The Charlevoix
COOK BOOK

The Charlevoix COOK BOOK

IT means the knowledge of Medea, and of Circe, and of Calypso, and of Helen, and of Rebekah, and of the Queen of Sheba. It means the knowledge of all herbs and fruits and balms and spices, and of all that is healing and sweet in fields and groves, and savory in meats. It means carefulness and inventiveness, watchfulness and willingness and readiness of appliance. It means much tasting and no wasting. It means the economy of our great-grandmothers and the science of modern chemists; and it means English thoroughness and French art and Arabian hospitality; and it means, in fine, that you are to be perfectly and always, "ladies" loaf givers.—*Ruskin.*

Charlevoix, Michigan
1907

BREAKFAST and SUPPER DISHES.

BAKED SUCCOTASH.

Cook one pint of dried Lima beans until they are very tender. Put a layer of the beans, one of canned corn and one of fine bread crumbs in a baking dish, seasoning with salt and pepper. Continue the layers in this way, having the last layer of crumbs. Pour on milk until you can see it around the edge, but not to cover. Cut small strips of fat salt pork and arrange around the edge so they radiate towards the center. Bake one hour in a moderate oven and brown on top.—Mrs. H. A. Putnam.

POP-OVERS.

One cup sweet milk, one cup flour, one egg, pinch of salt, one teaspoonful baking powder. Beat well and put a tablespoonful of the batter in each small tin.—Mrs. Grace Hyers.

BEATEN BISCUIT.

One quart flour, one heaping tablespoonful lard, one teaspoonful salt, enough milk to make very stiff. Beat until the dough snaps.—Mrs. Christy.

TOMATO GRAVY.

Put one tablespoonful of butter in a saucepan and when hot add one cup tomato (fresh or canned). When boiling sprinkle in one quarter teaspoonful soda. Stir two tablespoonfuls of flour smooth with a bowl of milk and cream and turn into the tomato. Cook until thick and smooth. Season with salt, pepper and butter. A nice supper dish.—Nellie Stites.

POTATO PANCAKE.

Two eggs, eight grated raw potatoes, four tablespoonfuls flour, one teaspoonful salt. Fry on well greased spider.

VELVET PANCAKES.

A delicate pancake, appetizing even in warm weather. Add a tablespoonful melted butter to one well beaten egg, one-half pint milk, one-half teaspoonful salt, one-half pint flour with which is sifted one teaspoonful cream of tartar, one-half teaspoonful soda disolved in one teaspoonful hot water. Beat well and bake at once on soap stone (or other) griddle.—Mrs. J. B. Thielen.

EGGS—BIRD'S NEST.

A pretty way to serve eggs is as follows: Separate the whites from the yolks, leaving the latter perfectly whole; beat the whites (with pinch of salt) until very stiff. Then form into mounds on a buttered baking dish. Make a tiny hollow in the top of each and place the yolks in them. Put in oven a few minutes until a delicate brown. Remove with buttered knife to hot platter. Add a dot of butter and dash of pepper to each and serve.—Mrs. J. Timmer.

LEMON BISCUITS.

Five cents worth oil of lemon, five cents worth baking ammonia, two cupfuls sweet milk, two and one-half cupfuls granulated sugar, one cupful lard. Soak the ammonia in one cup of the milk over night. When ready to bake beat two eggs in the remaining cupful of milk, then add the sugar, lard and lemon, then the milk and ammonia (which must be dissolved) and flour to make quite a stiff dough. Roll out and bake like cookies.—Mrs. F. E. Cartier.

GRAHAM GEMS.

One and one-half cups sour milk, one egg, five tablespoonfuls syrup, one teaspoonful soda. Thicken with graham flour.—Mrs. W. W. Srigley.

GEMS.

Either graham, whole wheat or corn meal may be used in making these gems. One egg beaten with half a teaspoonful of salt. One large stirring spoon of melted butter or other shortening, One-fourth teacup of sugar, one-half cup of wheat flour, one tea cup of sour milk in which stir a level teaspoonful of soda, add flour or meal enough to make a batter, not too stiff. This makes a dozen gems.—Mrs. H. S. Harsha.

GRAHAM GEMS.

One level cup graham flour, and two level cups of cold water. A little salt. Stir the water into the flour until there are no lumps. This quantity will fiill three sets of irons with a tablespoonful in each. The irons must be smoking hot, and then well greased. Bake in a hot oven about twenty minutes. If one part of the oven is hotter than another change the irons around so they will bake evenly. When done turn out on a plate with the top of the gems turned down, or they will steam and be soft.—Mrs. O. D. Wood.

OATMEAL GEMS.

Put two cups of rolled oats in a dish, add one and one-half cups sour milk and let it soak over night. In the morning add two teaspoonfuls melted butter, one-third cup of sugar, one egg, one teaspoonful soda, one good cup of flour and a little salt. Beat well. Can be baked in a loaf if desired and is nice cold.—Mrs. John Burns.

TEA ROLLS.

Scald three pints of milk; while hot put in one cup of butter and one cup of sugar. When cool add six quarts of sifted flour and one cup of soft yeast. Stir until smooth. Let stand over night to rise. Mold or knead the whole and let stand until about noon; when it is rolled out about one-half inch thick cut with small tin, one-half is folded upon the other, a small piece of butter being put in between. Let rise in a cool place until about four o'clock then bake in a hot oven for tea.—Mrs. Mattie Priest.

PARKER HOUSE CORN ROLLS.

One and one-fourth cups of white flour, three-fourths cup corn meal, four teaspoons baking powder, one-half teaspoon salt, one tablespoon of sugar, two tablespoons butter, one egg, three-fourths cup milk. Chop butter in with a knife. Beat egg. Add one-half cup milk and add to the dry ingredients to make a soft dough that can be handled. Add more milk if necessary. Turn on a floured board, toss lightly and roll out to one-half inch, but with a round cutter. Put a piece of butter the size of a pea in the center and fold so that the edges touch. Put on buttered tins. Rub the top with milk and bake in a quick oven twelve or fifteen minutes.—Mrs. C. L. Gonser.

MERRILL BREAD.

Scald one-half cup of flour, one-half cup of sugar and one scant half cup of salt with one quart of boiling water (I use potato water). When cool add one cake and a half of yeast that has been well soaked in water. Let this first part be ready, then cook about six or eight good sized potatoes, drain, mash and add one quart of boiling water and one quart of cold water. When cool enough mix with the first part and set in a warm place to rise. Allow one cup to a loaf and mix into a hard loaf without sponging at all; let rise, mold into loaves and bake in a quick oven.—Mrs. Rose Taylor.

CHEESE STRAWS.

Put one-half pound of sifted flour into a mixing bowl. Make a hollow in the center and put in it four ounces of butter, two of cheese, one egg, a pinch of red pepper and one gill of milk. Mix well together and roll out to the thickness of one eighth inch, cut in strips one-quarter of an inch wide and four inches long. Bake in a moderate oven until a light brown in color. Serve either hot or cold.—Mrs. J. B. Parsons.

ROLLS.

On baking day save enough dough for a large pan of rolls. Mix in two tablespoons shortening and the same of sugar. Knead all well together. Let it rise in dish and keep it chopped down as fast as it rises. About two or three hours before baking roll out and cut with round cutter and put in butter that has been melted. Fold together and place in pan close together. Let rise well and bake in a hot oven.—Mrs. P. D. Campbell.

PARKER HOUSE ROLLS.

One quart sweet milk boiled, when cool add flour to make batter and one yeast cake. When light add one-half cup butter, one cup sugar. Mix soft and let rise again. Roll out and cut with cookie cutter. Butter the top and fold together in a long roll. Let it rise very light. This will make about seventy rolls.—Mrs. Wright.

PLAIN MUFFINS.

One egg well beaten, a tablespoon of butter and a tablespoon of sugar, with a teaspoon of salt, all beaten until very light. One cup of milk, three of sifted flour and three teaspoonfuls of baking powder.—Mrs. J. B. Thielen.

LIGHT MUFFINS.

Two eggs, one cup sweet milk, a little salt, two tablespoons sugar, two tablespoons melted butter, two teaspoons baking powder. Flour for a stiff batter.—Mrs. R. B. Armstrong.

CORNMEAL MUFFINS.

Cream together one-half cup of sugar, and one tablespoon of butter. Add one egg,one cup of milk, one and one-half teaspoons baking powder and flour enough to make a thin batter. Then stir in enough corn meal to make of the proper consistency.—Mrs. A. S. Burnett.

MUFFINS.

Three cups flour, two heaping teaspoons baking powder, a little salt, two tablespoonfuls sugar. Sift all together, Two beaten eggs, one and one-half cups sweet milk. Melt one tablespoonful of butter and add last.—Mrs. B. Hartsig.

ONE-EGG MUFFINS.

One egg, two tablespoonfuls butter and lard melted, one-half teaspoonful salt, one cup milk, two and one-half cups flour, two and one-half teaspoonfuls baking powder.—Miss Geiken.

MUFFINS.

One-half cup melted butter (scant), one cup sweet milk, two and one-half cups flour, one egg, a pinch of salt, two teaspoonfuls baking powder. Make as stiff as cup cake.—Mrs. Grace Hyers.

RICE FRITTERS.

One cup cooked rice, one-half cup cold meat chopped fine, one egg, salt, dash pepper. Make in balls and roll in cracker crumbs. Fry in butter or part meat drippings. This makes enough for four.—Mrs. L. E. Bailey.

CREAM MUFFINS.

Two teaspoonfuls baking powder, one-half teaspoonful salt, one pint sifted flour; two eggs; one-half cup sweet milk, one-third cup of butter. Mix baking powder and salt with flour; beat the yolks of the eggs, add to them the milk and stir into the flour. Then stir in the butter, softened, and lastly the egg whites, well beaten. Fill greased muffin-pans two-thirds full and bake about fifteen minutes in a very hot oven.—Mrs. Glasford.

MUFFINS.

One-fourth cup sugar, one-fourth cup butter, one cup sweet milk, two cups flour, two teaspoons baking powder, salt; bake twenty minutes.—Miss Mabelle Buttars.

GREEN CORN MUFFINS.

Cut the rows of corn down through the middle and scrape out the pulp with a knife. To two cups of corn add one saltspoon of salt, one tablespoonful of butter, the beaten yolks of three eggs, two cups of milk, three cups of flour, in which two teaspoonfuls of baking powder have been sifted. Mix thoroughly, add carefully the whites of eggs, beaten stiff. Have pop-over irons heated and greased, half fill with the mixture. Bake in a quick oven for half an hour and eat at once.—Harriet G. West.

GRAHAM MUFFINS.

Two cups graham flour, two tablespoonfuls melted butter, one tablespoonful sugar, one egg, one cup of milk, two rather heaping teaspoons baking powder. Beat well together, sugar and egg, add milk, then graham flour, then melted butter, baking powder last. Drop into warm muffin tins. Bake twenty minutes or half an hour.—Mrs. Fred Smith.

GRAHAM MUFFINS.

Into a bowl put one and one-half pints of Graham, half a cupful of sugar and a teaspoonful of salt. Into a sieve put half a pint of flour, a teaspoonful of soda and two of cream of tartar and sift on the material in the bowl. Mix all thoroughly while dry and add two well-beaten eggs and a pint of milk. Fill muffin cups about two-thirds to the top and bake in a quick oven.—Mrs. R. W. Paddock.

SHREDDED WHEAT BISCUIT WITH STRAWBERRIES.

Prepare berries as for ordinary serving. Warm biscuit in oven before using. Cut or crush oblong cavity in top of biscuit to form basket. Fill the cavity with berries and serve with cream or milk. Sweeten to taste. Peaches, blackberries, raspberries, blueberries, pineapple, bananas and other fruit, fresh or preserved, can be served with Shredded Wheat Biscuit in the same way.

DELICIOUS SANDWICHES.

Boil as many eggs as may be required for twenty minutes, then plunge in cold water, remove the shells and separate the whites from the yolks. Chop whites to the finest possible mince. Rub the yolks to a paste with a little melted butter and flavor generously with anchovy sauce. Add a few drops of lemon juice and cayenne to taste. Lastly stir in the minced white. Cut white bread, twenty-four hours old, into very thin slices, butter and spread with the paste; lay one slice over the other and chop into triangles with a sandwich cutter; dip the edges into finely chopped parsley. —Mrs. Robert Davidson.

SHREDDED WHEAT BISCUIT FOR BREAKFAST.

Warm the biscuit in the oven to restore crispness; don't burn; pour hot milk over it, dipping the milk over it until the shreds are swollen; then pour a little cream over the top of the biscuit; or serve with cold milk or cream, according to individual taste.

GREEN PEPPERS WITH SALMON FILLING.

One can of salmon flaked, one-quarter teaspoonful salt, two tablespoonfuls of chopped gherkins, two tablespoonfuls of chopped olives, two tablespoonfuls of chopped capers, Mayonnaise dressing and green peppers. Remove seeds, membrane and stem end from peppers and soak in salt water. Mix gherkins, olives, capers and salt with salmon; add enough Mayonnaise to hold it together; fill peppers, garnish and serve.—Mrs. J. A. Noble.

SHREDDED WHEAT OYSTER, MEAT OR VEGETABLE PATTIES.

Cut oblong cavity in top of biscuit, remove top carefully and all inside shreds, forming a shell. Sprinkle with salt and pepper, put small pieces of butter in bottom and fill the shell with drained, picked and washed oysters. Season with additional salt and pepper. Replace top of biscuit over oysters, then bits of butter on top. Place in a covered pan and bake in a moderate oven. Pour oyster liquor or cream sauce over it. Shell fish, vegetables or meats may also be used.

SOUPS.

MEATLESS TOMATO SOUP.

One quart tomatoes, one quart water, stew until soft; add one teaspoonful soda, allow to effervesce, add one quart boiling milk, salt, butter and pepper to taste, with a little rolled cracker. Boil a few minutes and serve. Enough for twelve persons.—Mrs. F. N. Chapel.

NOODLE SOUP.

A nice marrow soup-bone weighing about two pounds, four quarts water boiled down to two quarts, seasoned with salt and pepper to suit the taste. Half a large cup of drippings, a pinch of salt (if drippings), a small half-cup of water; work in all the flour you can, roll thin, cut in strips half inch wide, drop in the broth and cook.—Mrs. A. Chamberlin.

POTAGE ST. GERMAIN.

Take a carrot, onion, stick of celery, two cloves and a green pepper, add one cup of dried peas, three pints of water; boil slowly three hours, strain and add a cup of cream; serve with slice of bread fried lightly in butter.

TOMATO SOUP.

One dozen ripe tomatoes, or one can of tomatoes. Cook in one quart of water; strain and add one pint of milk or cream, a lump of butter the size of an egg, salt to taste, one teaspoonful flour for the thickening. Serve hot.—A. Rodger.

POTATO SOUP.

One quart of milk, eight potatoes, one tablespoonful butter, one stalk of celery, one onion. Boil milk with onions and celery, boil potatoes and mash fine, add boiling milk after straining out the onion and celery. Add butter, salt and pepper to taste. Miss K. L. Meech.

MULLIGATAWNEY SOUP.

To one quart of chicken stock add one teacup of chopped chicken, one teacup of bread crumbs, put through a colander; then take two hard-boiled eggs, chop the whites very fine, mash the yolks soft with a big spoonful of butter; stir all together, salt and pepper to taste; add, the last thing, one cup of sweet cream and a tiny bit of parsley.—Mrs. H. Lee Iddings.

CORN SOUP.

One pint of hot water, one pint of grated green corn or one can of corn, one quart of milk, one heaping tablespoon of flour, two tablespoons of butter, one slice of onion, salt and pepper to taste. Cook the corn in water for thirty minutes. Let the milk and onion come to a boil. Mix together the flour and butter, and when perfectly smooth stir into the boiling milk and let it boil a few minutes. Take out onion and add the corn. Season to taste. If canned corn is used it should be strained before putting into the milk.—Miss L. P. Averill.

CELERY SOUP.

One head of celery cut in small pieces, put into a pint of boiling water which has been salted. Cook until very soft, wash it in the water in which it was boiled. Cook one tablespoonful of chopped onion in one pint of milk in a double boiler fifteen or twenty minutes and add the celery to it. Put all through a strainer and put it on to boil again. Rub one tablespoonful of butter in one tablespoonful of flour until smooth and stir into the boiling soup. Season with salt and pepper to taste. Serve very hot with a little whipped cream on each plate.

CREAM CELERY SOUP.

Chop one head of celery and cook in one pint each of water and soup stock. Add one-half pint of rich milk or cream and one tablespoonful of flour rubbed into one tablespoonful of butter. Season with salt and pepper. Heat again and serve at once. Mrs. A. L. Coulter.

MEATLESS BEAN SOUP.

Parboil one pint beans, drain off the water, add fresh, let boil in plenty of water till perfectly tender, season with pepper, salt and butter. When done skim out half the beans, leaving the broth with the remaining half in the kettle; pour through the colander, mashing the beans to take out the skins, put back in the kettle and add one cup milk and a dozen crackers broken up; let come to a boil and serve. To the beans taken out add salt or salt pork, pepper, molasses to taste and water to cover and bake in the oven for supper.—Mrs. F. N. Chapel.

CABBAGE SOUP.

One quart of stock, half of small head of cabbage shredded fine, one very small onion, one bay leaf, salt, pepper; boil one hour. When ready to serve add half a cup cream. —Mrs. Partridge.

FISH.

DEVILED SHRIMP.

Open a pint can of shrimp and put them into cold water an hour before using. Heat together in the chafing dish two tablespoons of butter and one of Worcestershire sauce, add to these one-fourth teaspoonful mustard, one-half teaspoonful salt. Lay the shrimp in this and when all is hot put in one teaspoonful minced parsley, six drops Tobasco sauce and the juice of a small lemon. Serve on toast. Lobster can be served in this way.—Mrs. O. A. Sears.

SALMON LOAF.

One can salmon, one cup sweet milk, one cup bread crumbs, one-third cup butter, one teaspoonful salt, one-half teaspoonful pepper, two eggs. Melt butter and beat the eggs before adding to the salmon. Bake in a buttered dish one-half hour.—Mrs. F. E. Cartier.

ESCALLOPED SALMON.

Put in baking dish a thin layer of salmon, season with pepper, salt and small pieces of butter, then a layer of cracker crumbs. Continue this way until you have the amount wanted. Last layer should be of crackers. Cover with milk and bake in a hot oven until thoroughly heated. Serve immediately.—Mrs. F. Butler.

SALMON LOAF.

Melt two tablespoonfuls butter in saucepan, add two eggs well beaten, two-thirds cup cracker crumbs, salt and pepper to taste, one can salmon (remove bone and skin), mix together well. Put in greased baking powder can (one pound can) and steam one hour. Remove from can while hot. Serve cold with hard boiled eggs, parsely and sliced lemon.

ROYAL SCOLLOP.

Two hard boiled eggs, one can salmon, two cups bread crumbs, two cups white sauce. White Sauce—Four tablespoonfuls butter, two tablespoonfuls flour, two cups hot milk. Salt and pepper to taste. Mash eggs fine with fork. Butter a baking dish and arrange food materials in layers—crumbs, fish, eggs and sauce—repeat, finish with crumbs on top. Bake until brown.—Mrs. O. E. Wilbur.

BAKED SALMON CREAM.

One small can salmon, one cup milk, one-fourth teaspoon salt, a dash of pepper, one small onion, sprig of parsley, two tablespoons butter, two tablespoons flour, one-half cup buttered cracker crumbs. Cook the milk, onion, parsley, salt and pepper together fifteen minutes. Strain. Melt the butter in sauce pan. Add flour. Mix well. Add the cooked milk and cook until thickens. Cover the bottom of small baking dish with half the salmon (this should be well picked to pieces) then half the sauce. Repeat and cover with the crumbs and bake till the crumbs are nicely browned.—Mrs. C. L. Gonser.

FISH TIMBALES.

One-half pound halibut or white fish, the whites of five eggs, one level teaspoonful salt, one-half pint soft bread crumbs, one gill milk, six tablespoons cream, one saltspoon white pepper. Boil milk and bread crumbs until a smooth paste. When cool put in the fish which has been put through the meat chopper twice. Add cream, salt and pepper and fold in the well beaten whites of the eggs. Grease small timbale molds. Put paper in bottom. Fill with the mixture, place in pan partly filled with hot water. bake twenty minutes. Serve with lobster, shrimp or oyster sauce. Garnish with mushroons, peas or serve plain.—Mrs. Susan L. Thomas.

CODFISH LUNCHEON DISH.

Line well-buttered bread tin with mashed potato and fill with creamed codfish. Then cover with potatoes, putting bits of butter on the top. Bake in quick oven forty-five minutes. Turn out to serve.—Mrs. Susan Louise Thomas.

CLAM CHOWDER.

Piece of butter size of egg, brown in soup kettle, add a medium sized onion. Chop fine. Small cup of salt pork, cut fine. One pint of sliced raw potatoes, cover with boiling water. Season with salt and pepper. Add contents of can of minced clams. One-half cup of cream.—Mrs. Iddings.

CODFISH OR SALMON BALLS.

One cup of fish shredded, one-half cup mashed potatoes, one tablespoon cream, one egg. Mash freshened fish with the potato. Then add egg, milk and salt. Use a spoon to make balls and drop from spoon into very hot lard. Much depends upon the frying.—Mrs. Susan L. Thomas.

TURBOT.

Take a whitefish, steam till tender, take out bones and sprinkle with salt and pepper. For Dressing—Heat a pint of milk and thicken with flour. When cool add two eggs, tablespoonful butter and season with onion and parsley. Put in baking dish a layer of fish and a layer of sauce till full. Cover the top with bread crumbs and bake a half hour. —Mrs. D. H. Fitch.

An oyster omelet, prepared in the chafing dish; that recommends itself for the Sunday night tea, is made in this wise: Cut in two a half pint of oysters, raw or cooked, and sprinkle with a half teaspoon of lemon juice and a half saltspoon of pepper. Beat three eggs, whites and yolks separately, adding the oysters and three scant tablespoons of oyster liquor or milk to the yolks. Put a tablespoonful of butter in the cutlet pan over the hot water pan, buttering the sides thoroughly. When hot pour in the beaten whites and then the yolks with the oysters. Do not stir, simply cut them in. Cover and cook twenty minutes. If desired, this may be turned spoonful by spoonful, or simply served from the chafing dish on hot plates.—Mrs. Sears.

BAKED OYSTERS.

Open one dozen large oysters, lay them in the deep shells, season with paprika. Lay a thin slice of raw bacon the same length as the oysters on top, with a piece of fresh butter. Place oysters in baking pan for about five minutes, and bake to a nice color. Dress on a hot platter, garnish with parsley and pieces of lemon.—Mrs. Noble.

SALMON LOAF.

One pound can of salmon, liquor drained off, two-thirds cup of bread crumbs, four eggs, four tablespoonfuls melted butter, a pinch of salt and dash of pepper. Mix salmon and butter together smooth, beat the eggs light and add to them the bread crumbs and other ingredients and thoroughly mix. Put in a buttered mold and steam one hour.

Dressing.—One cup of milk, one scant tablespoonful of corn starch, one egg, a little salt and the least bit of red pepper. Scald milk, thicken with the corn starch, cook a moment then add the egg well beaten and cook an instant longer. Strain and add the liquor from the fish, put in a small piece of butter and pour over the loaf when ready to serve.—Mrs. Fred W. Mayne.

MEATS.

CHICKEN IN MUSHROOMS.

Boil two chickens till tender, cut them in small pieces as you would for salad. Take one can of mushrooms and boil them in their own liquor for five minutes, cut them into small pieces and mix with the chicken. Make a cream sauce as follows: One teaspoonful flour to a cup of cream (this amount of chicken will probably take three cups of cream). Pour this over the chicken, season with pepper and salt. Put bread crumbs and small bits of butter on top. Bake three-quarters of an hour in a quick oven.—Mrs. H. L. Iddings.

CREAMED CHICKEN.

Boil until tender one good sized chicken. Remove all bone, cut or pick in pieces. Make a gravy of liquor in which it was boiled, thicken with flour, add a pint of cream and butter size of a walnut or part milk may be used with more butter. Chop very fine, some parsley and onions, stir about one tablespoonful of each into the gravy, season with pepper and salt, let boil but do not burn. Cover the bottom of baking dish (buttered) with bread or cracker crumbs, then a layer of chicken, on this a layer of gravy, alternating until the dish is full, covering top with crumbs. Bake twenty minutes. Veal may be used instead of chicken.—Mrs. Rebecca Lewis. Excellent.

BAKED SWEETBREADS.

Put cold water on sweet-breads after removing the membranes. Let them stand for a couple of hours, then parboil until tender. Take out all veins, strings, etc. and break into good sized pieces. Roll in beaten white of egg and then in cracker crumbs. Place in a baking pan, dot with small pieces of butter and bake in moderate oven half an hour. Serve on toast.—Miss L. P. Averill.

VEAL AND RICE LOAF.

Large cup meat, put through meat chopper. one-half small onion, two cups boiled rice (very dry), two tablespoonfuls of gravy, or little melted butter, salt and pepper. Make in loaf and bake twenty minutes.—Mrs. Thirza Miller.

BEEFSTEAK AND MUSHROOMS.

Put into a sauce pan one ounce of butter, a small onion chopped fine, a little ground sage and thyme, and put it over the fire. When hot shake in two tablespoons of flour and when it becomes brown put in one gill of water and let it boil for half an hour, slowly. Then add three tablespoons of beef stock and a little suet. Put in one can of mushrooms, let it boil ten minutes. Pour this over a nicely broiled beefsteak.—Miss L. P. Averill.

ESCALLOPED CHICKEN.

Cut up or chop cold chicken in small pieces, put these in a buttered baking dish. Sprinkle with flour and season with pepper, chopped parsley, salt. Moisten with cream or milk. If the latter is used add butter, and remnant of gravy. Take cold boiled rice, heat, adding a little milk to moisten. Spread over the chicken about an inch in thickness. Bread crumbs should be used last as the rice hardens if left exposed, put in bits of butter and bake thirty minutes.

BEEF LOAF.

For one and one-half pounds of beef allow one-fourth pound of salt pork. Run these through the meat chopper together then add one beaten egg, five tablespoonfuls of cracker crumbs, three tablespoonfuls of milk. Mix well and pack in a baking dish. Pour one-half cup of boiling water over meat. Bake in a moderate oven for about one hour.—Mrs. E. A. Burnett.

CROQUETTES.

This holds good for any croquettes you would like to make. Grind through cutter and to two cupfuls of veal cooked and seasoned, add one cupful of gravy or stock, or sauce supreme. Mix while warm and pour on platter to cool. Put where it will get perfectly cool. Take a rounding tablespoonful for each. Put some bread crumbs on the board, let them dry for twenty minutes, then roll croquettes in beaten eggs. Be sure to get the egg on the ends as well as on the sides. Now roll in the crumbs on the board and be sure to have plenty of crumbs. Let stand to dry about one-half hour before you use them. Have the fat smoking hot and immerse the croquettes just long enough to brown on outside. Then you have a crisp outside and a creamy inside. —Mrs. Benton.

TOMALE LOAF.

One and one-fourth pounds of lean beef, two medium sized onions, one long red pepper, one small section of garlic. Cut these in small pieces. Add one and a quarter quarts of hot water and one-half can of tomatoes, and boil together until the meat is tender. Take the meat out and chop, but not very fine. Strain the rest through a colander, mashing as much of the onion and tomatoes as will go through, (throwing the rest away). Then add the chopped meat, one and one-fourth quarts of water, one-half tablespoonful salt, one-half teaspoon red pepper, one tablespoon Gebhardt's Eagle Chili powder. Thirty drops of Tobasco sauce. When thoroughly heated, before it boils, add slowly one and three-fourths cups yellow cornmeal, and let it boil slowly for three-fourths of an hour,—stir all the time to keep it from burning. Five minutes before taking off the fire add one pint of small green olives. If it gets too stiff add a little more water.—Miss Edmundson.

SAUCE SUPREME.

Put in a saucepan a tablespoonful of melted butter and two level tablespoonfuls of flour. Put over the fire and stir the flour and butter together. If you want it brown it will be necessary to brown the butter, then stir in the flour. Then put in one cup of milk and stir till smooth. When sauce is cooled add a teaspoonful of salt.—Mrs. L. E. Benton.

MEAT LOAF.

One pound each of chopped veal, beef and lean pork, one tablespoonful butter, salt, pepper, two eggs, one cup milk, one cup hot water. Make in loaf and roll in bread crumbs. Bake one and one-half hours. Add one cup rich milk to liquor and make gravy and pour over top.—Winnifred Rice.

FRITTADILLA.

One pint finely chopped cold meat of different kinds. One pint bread crumbs. One tablespoonful onion, chopped fine. One tablespoonful chopped parsley. Salt and pepper to taste. Soak bread crumbs and drain. Put one tablespoonful butter in spider, when melted drop in onion for three minutes. Then put in bread crumbs and meat. Heat all through. Mix all together with two well beaten eggs. Make into little pats. Fry in butter until brown.—Harriet G. West.

VEAL LOAF.

Two pounds veal chopped fine, one-fourth pound pork, two eggs well beaten, one cup cracker crumbs, one cup sweet milk, one tablespoonful salt. Bake in slow oven one and one-half hours. Baste often.—Mrs. J. L. Crane.

VEAL LOAF.

One pound raw veal chopped fine, one egg, one-half cup fine bread crumbs, butter size of walnut, one tablespoonful milk, two teaspoonfuls salt, one-fourth teaspoonful pepper. Mix solid and pack into a one pound baking powder can, placing cover on, and boil three hours.—Mrs. F. E. Lewis.

VENISON.

Take a haunch of venison, cover with water and boil until tender. Draw off the water. Put one-half pound butter with salt and pepper into the kettle over a moderate fire turning the meat to let it brown on all sides. Venison cooked in this way is delicious.—From Kentucky.

BAKED VEAL CUTLET.

One and one-half pounds veal cutlet laid in a well buttered roasting pan. Pour over a cup of water then spread a dressing made as follows:

Two cups bread crumbs, two onions chopped fine, two well beaten eggs. Butter size of an egg, salt and pepper. Mix well, cover and bake one-half hour. Remove the lid and brown.—Mrs. B. W. Miller.

ROAST DUCK.

Parboil the duck for about fifteen minutes. Stuff with one cup of bread crumbs, one cup of mashed potato, one sour apple with a little salt pork chipped very fine, pepper and salt to taste. Roast one hour then cover the breast with slices of onion that have been boiled until tender. Baste frequently until duck is done and onions a golden brown.—Miss L. P. Averill.

HASH.

One cupful of tender cooked meat, chopped fine, two cupfuls of hot mashed potatoes, one-half teaspoonful of salt, one-half saltspoonful of pepper. Mix till there are no lumps. Put three tablespoonfuls of hot water into a spider, melt in it one tablespoonful of butter or drippings, put in the hash, let it simmer slowly till it has absorbed the water and formed a brown crust; do not stir; fold over as you would an omelet and turn on a hot dish.

RAGOUT OF BEEF.

Take about six pounds of a boiling piece of beef (or more if there are many bones). Cut gashes in the meat, and stuff them with one-half pound fat salt pork, cut into bits. Put into a vessel with a tight cover, one tin can of tomatoes, two or three onions, cut up, one-half dozen cloves, one stick cinnamon, broken; and a little whole black pepper. Place the meat on the other ingredients, and pour over them one-half cup of vinegar and one cup of water; cover tightly and bake in a moderate oven; cook slowly four or five hours, and, when about half done, salt to taste. When done, take out the meat, strain the gravy through a colander, and thicken with flour. —Mrs. F. N. Chapel.

CARROT STEW.

Cold or fresh meat can be used. Put piece of butter in sauce pan, add meat and brown on both sides. Add onion, one bay leaf and medium-sized carrot; salt. Add a little water and let stew for an hour. When ready to serve, thicken it. Place stew in center of platter. Garnish with carrots, which should be cut round.—Mrs. Partridge.

CHICKEN BALLS.

One cup of chopped chicken to the white of one egg makes four balls. One-half teaspoon of salt, pepper to taste. Mix salt, pepper, egg and chicken together and shape into balls. Cook in boiling hot water four minutes.—Mrs. Merriam.

DRESSING—For Stewed, Fried or Baked Chicken.

One tablespoon butter, one tablespoon flour, three-fourths cup of chicken stock, three-fourths cup of sweet cream and one-half cup of shredded almonds.—Mrs. Merriam.

VEAL LOAF.

Two pounds of nice lean veal, one-half pound of fat salt pork, three eggs, three Boston crackers rolled, one nutmeg, salt and pepper to taste. Veal and pork to be chopped like sausage meat. Bake slowly for two and one-half hours.—Mrs. F. J. Meech.

In preparing crust for game pie, cut dough into biscuits, lay on top of fowl and bake.—Mrs. A. L. Coulter.

ESCALLOPED CHICKEN.

Stew a chicken until very tender and separate the meat into fine pieces. Butter a baking dish; then place a layer of cracker crumbs, salt, pepper and butter flakes, then a layer of chicken within the dish alternately until the dish is filled. Make a dressing of stock and cream. Cover the top with fine bread crumbs and flakes of butter. Bake forty-five minutes, moistening when dry with the dressing.—Mrs. Merriam.

BEEFSTEAK. (Fit for a King.)

With a sharp knife remove fat, and all stringy substances which prevent the steak from lying flat while cooking. Pound steak with smooth wooden mallet, or its equivalent, crosswise the grain. Have a hot fire with plenty of coals. Put enough suet in an iron spider to grease it well, adding more as necessity requires. When the spider is real hot, put in one or two pieces, according to your heat (do not cook enough at one time to cool the spider), count ten and turn, lifting with a knife and fork, repeating until cooked to suit the taste, rare or well done; lift from the spider carefully, placing on hot platter, turn on hot suet, salt and butter, which will make a rich gravy. Serve on hot plates. The secret of a good steak is, not to let the juice get started when cooking. Never put on salt until the steak is cooked. (Venison may be cooked the same.)—Mary E. Heston.

COLD MEATS.

PRESSED VEAL.

Cook three pounds of veal until it falls from the bone; chop rather coarsely, and season well. Boil the liquor to a pint and add one-half box of gelatine dissolved in cold water. Line a mold with slices of three hard boiled eggs, then put in the chopped meat and pour the liquor over it. Place in a cold place to set. Remove from the mold to a bed of lettuce leaves to serve.—Mrs. D. H. Fitch.

POMO SANDWICHES.

Cut the bread into very thin slices and spread with butter; spread with mayonnaise dressing, and place very thin slices of apples between the sandwiches. These are very nice.—Mrs. F. M. Graham.

PIG'S HEAD CHEESE.

Have the head split in two. Cut off and throw away the end of the nose, the jaw bone with teeth, and cut out eyes and brain. Cut off ears for convenience in cleaning. Singe the pieces carefully, and then wash and scrape and clean through four or five hot waters till perfectly clean, and put on to boil slowly. A beef tongue added to it makes it nicer as it is apt to be too fat for many. The pigs' feet can also be added if desired to increase the quantity.

Skim as any scum rises and keep covered with water; when boiled so that the flesh leaves the bones, take it from the water with a skimmer into a large wooden bowl. Pick over carefully to remove every particle of bone, and either chop the meat coarsely or pick it up with the fingers. Add salt and pepper to taste and sage, as desired. Spread a cloth over the colander, or steamer; put the meat in, fold cloth closely over it, lay a weight on it so that it may press the whole surface equally (flat irons or a stone on top of a plate the right size, answer nicely). If the meat is to be lean, use a heavy weight; if fat, a lighter one. When cold, remove and keep in a cold place.—Mrs. F. N. Chapel.

BEEF LOAF.

Three and one-half pounds of the round steak, one cup rolled crackers, one cup milk, two eggs well beaten. Salt to suit the taste.—Mrs. George F. Brown.

PRESSED MEAT.

One pound smoked ham, two pounds veal, juice of one lemon, one teaspoonful of prepared mustard, salt if needed. Cook meat in just enough water to cover. Do not have over a pint when done. Grind or chop coarsely. Add lemon and other ingredients with the stock and press. It is best prepared the day before using. —Mrs. Cruickshank.

BEEF LOAF.

Two pounds of beef, chopped with one-half pound of lean fresh pork. Have a large mixing bowl in which beat two eggs. Add a level tablespoon of salt, one-half cup melted butter, three cups of cold water, a trace of pepper, nutmeg and cloves, and a pint of cracker crumbs. Then put in the chopped meat and mix thoroughly. Press into a loaf in a buttered baking pan and bake two hours, basting occasionally with hot water.—Mrs. H. S. Harsha.

A chicken loaf may be made the same way, excluding the pork.

HORSE RADISH TABLE SAUCE.

Half pint of grated horse radish, one teaspoonful of salt, one-half teaspoonful of mustard, vinegar to cover well, half a cupful of good thick cream, either sweet or sour.—Mrs. A. Chamberlin.

Cold chicken chopped very fine, mixed with hot cream and a little salt, makes excellent filling for sandwiches.

SALADS.

FRUIT SALAD.

Make a dressing by boiling one cup of water and one-fourth cup of sugar for five minutes, then put away to cool. Beat the yolk of one egg until thick and creamy, add to it four tablespoons of thick sweet cream, then add the syrup and the juice from the fruit which you have prepared for salad. Use one banana sliced, one cup of diced pineapple, four fresh peaches, one pint of raspberries; arrange the fruit in a pyramid form, and pour the dressing over it.—Mrs. J. B. Parsons.

POTATO SALAD.

Take some cold boiled potato sliced thin, three hard boiled eggs chopped, and one small onion chopped, prepare in salad bowl; first layer of potato, then a layer of eggs, sprinkle over them a little of the onion, pepper and salt.

For Dressing.—Take the yolk of a raw egg, stir into it one-half a teaspoonful made mustard, slowly beat into it three tablespoonfuls sweet cream, add one tablespoonful strong vinegar and the white of one egg beaten to a stiff froth. If needed for supper, make at noon time. A little chopped celery or flakes of cold boiled salmon may be added.—Mrs. S. J. Alcox.

TOMATO JELLY.

Use one quart can tomatoes, one teaspoon of salt, one sliced onion, one-quarter teaspoon paprika, juice of one-half lemon, six whole cloves, one small blade mace, a sprig of parsley, one inch of bay leaf, three-quarters of box of gelatine, three-quarters of cup of water.

Put tomato into sauce pan, adding all other ingredients, except cold water and lemon juice. Let simmer twenty to twenty-five minutes. While hot strain through seive and add gelatine soaked in three-quarters of cup of water. Stir until gelatine is dissolved, then add lemon juice. Strain into cold mould and set on ice until firm. Serve on lettuce leaves with Mayonnaise dressing.—Winnifred Rice.

ASPARAGUS SALAD.

Asparagus tips, fresh if you can get them; if not, canned ones. Arranged on individual plates of lettuce. Mayonnaise dressing poured over it.—Mrs. Fred Smith.

APPLE SALAD.

Three cups chopped apples, one cup nuts for dressing. Mix together in a bowl, one tablespoon flour, one tablespoon sugar, one-half teaspoon salt, on-third teaspoon mustard, and a little cayenne pepper. Beat yolks of two eggs and mix smooth with dry ingredients, then pour on slowly two-thirds of a cup of weak vinegar that has been brought to a boiling point. Set bowl over boiling water and let cook until thick, then add a little butter, and when ready to serve, one-half cup sweet cream. Serve with whipped cream.—Lillian Compton.

SALAD PICKLE.

Sprinkle one dozen medium-sized cucumbers with one cup of salt—the cucumbers to be peeled and sliced as for table use. Let stand over night. Wash and drain most thoroughly. Place in a stone jar and pour over cold, one quart of vinegar, one cup of olive oil, one ounce of white mustard seed, one-half ounce each of black mustard seed and celery seed. Keep in a cool place.—Mrs. Archibald Buttars.

SALAD DRESSING FOR CABBAGE (My Own.)

One cup of sweet cream, one-half cup of sugar, one-quarter teaspoon of mustard, dissolved in a little hot water; one-quarter teaspoonful of salt, two teaspoonfuls of vinegar. Add hard boiled eggs sliced.—Mrs. E. H. Green.

SALMON SALAD.

One can salmon, one-third small cabbage, two stalks celery, two tablespoons lemon juice and little grated rind, one tablespoon vinegar, one teaspoon salt, one-third teaspoon pepper. Make cup full of salad dressing, pick salmon to pieces with fork. Add lemon juice, vinegar, and put in cool place two hours. When ready to use, mix all together with dressing. In summer, use lettuce in place of cabbage. —Mrs. F. Crane.

POTATO SALAD.

Mix nice salad dressing of one teaspoonful of salt, a little pepper, two tablespoonfuls of finely cut crisp parsley, one onion, about two teaspoonfuls, with four teaspoonfuls of salad oil or butter. To this add eight tablespoonfuls of vinegar; slice two quarts of cold boiled potatoes; have these sliced not very thin; pour over the dressing and let them stand half an hour before serving.

DRESSING FOR CABBAGE.

Three eggs, one-half cup of vinegar. Salt and pepper. Put in a sauce pan and stir until boiling. Add sugar and mustard to your taste. One cup of cream.—A. Rodger.

CHICKEN SALAD.

Four eggs, one tablespoonful of mixed mustard, one teaspoonful of salt, one tablespoonful of hard butter, two-thirds cup of vinegar, four tablespoonfuls olive oil, two-thirds cup sweet cream. Beat the yolks and whites of eggs separately, into that beat the oil slowly. Mix all ingredients in an earthen dish, excepting the cream, and set on stove. Cook until as thick as pound cake. When cold, add the cream, stirring well, and pour over the chicken one hour before eating.—Mrs. N. A. Shores.

APPLE SALAD.

Two cups chopped apples, one cup chopped nuts, both fine. Season with a little cinnamon.

Dressing.—One egg well beaten, add six tablespoonfuls sugar, one-fourth tablespoonful mustard dissolved in three of water, one tablespoonful vinegar added slowly; cook until proper thickness. Remove from fire and add one tablespoonful butter, stir until dissolved; when cold, add one-half cup of whipped cream or three tablespoonfuls milk. Mix with the apples and nuts and garnish with whipped cream.—Mrs. Shores.

BEET SALAD.

Boil six beets until tender, peel, chop fine, add salt. Then make dressing of one egg, pinch mustard, one-fourth cup granulated sugar, three-fourths cup vinegar; boil until smooth. Pour this over the beets; just before serving cut in slices cold boiled eggs and place on top.—Mrs. John Ackart.

POTATO SALAD.

Cut cold boiled potatoes into small cubes, cucumbers and onions into small cubes or very thin slices. Add the following dressing and toss lightly together:

One teaspoonful salt, dash of pepper, six tablespoonfuls vinegar, two tablespoonfuls sugar, yolks of two eggs; beaten fine with flour and one-half teaspoonful mustard. Stir into the boiling vinegar, remove from fire, add butter size of egg and when cool add one cup of whipped cream. —Margaret Frazier.

POTATO SALAD.

One cupful of boiling vinegar, one heaping teaspoonful of flour, three tablespoonfuls of oil or butter, three tablespoonfuls of sugar, three teaspoonfuls of prepared mustard, one teaspoonful salt, one teaspoonful ground celery, a pinch of cayenne, and black pepper to taste. Mix all thoroughly together and pour slowly into the boiling vinegar. Let simmer until it thickens. Have the potatoes ready, chopped or sliced, cold. One onion and hard boiled eggs added to potatoes is an improvement. Pour dressing over potatoes and garnish with hard boiled eggs.—Mrs. A. M. Burdick.

CELERY SALAD.

Five potatoes, one-half dozen eggs, small bunch celery chopped; salt to taste. Use mayonnaise dressing to put over salad.

Mayonnaise Dressing.—One-half teacup vinegar in sauce pan and let boil. Yolks of four eggs, one tablespoon flour, one tablespoon cream, one tablespoon salt, lump of butter, one tablespoon white mustard, white pepper to suit taste. —Miss Juanita Felts.

POTATO SALAD DRESSING.

One-half pint vinegar, one teaspoonful mustard, one teaspoonful celery seed, one teaspoonful curry powder, a little pepper and salt, one-half onion and two tablespoonfuls sugar. Boil and strain and add well-beaten yolks of ten eggs and one tablespoonful butter. When ready to use, add cream, potatoes and boiled eggs, one and one-half lemon chopped. Can be put in glass jar and will keep.—Mrs. O. D. Hammond.

SALAD DRESSING.

One-half cup vinegar, one-half cup water, piece of butter, one-half teaspoonful flour, three tablespoonfuls sugar, one teaspoonful dry mustard, salt and pepper, two eggs. Boil. Add two cups sweet cream.—Mrs. W. J. Stevenson.

FRUIT SALAD DRESSING.

One whole egg, yolks of four, two-thirds cup of sugar, one-half teaspoonful mustard, one-fourth teaspoonful salt, one-half teaspoonful butter. Mix mustard and sugar and beat with the eggs. When well beaten, add one-half cup of vinegar and two-thirds cup of sweet cream. Cook in a double boiler until it begins to thicken. Serve with toasted crackers.—Mrs. O. D. Wood.

WHITE DRESSING FOR WALDORF SALAD.

Take two-thirds cup of sweet cream, two teaspoonfuls sugar, one teaspoonful salt, cayenne to taste, two teaspoonfuls butter. Stand the little pan you make it in in a sauce pan of boiling water. If it is not fairly thick, add half a teaspoonful of corn starch mixed with cold water. Boil one minute. Arrange the lettuce on individual plates. Put about two tablespoonfuls of chopped apples on the lettuce and pour the dressing over it. I always use chopped nuts with this and candied cherries on top. Apples and celery with this dressing makes a nice salad.—Mrs. Fred Smith.

TOMATO JELLY SALAD.

To make a very delicious and pretty salad. Drain the juice from one quart of tomatoes, season well with salt and pepper, and heat to the boiling point. Soak one box gelatine in cold water, pour the boiling tomato juice over it and stir until dissolved. Strain, put in small cups wet with cold water, and place on ice to harden. Serve with dressing on crisp lettuce leaves.—Cora Lee Bentley.

BANANA SALAD.

Peel and cut bananas in half. Roll each piece in mayonnaise dressing, then in chopped nuts. Place on individual plates of lettuce with two or three candied cherries.—Mrs. Fred Smith.

SALAD DRESSING.

Two eggs, well beaten, four tablespoonfuls of sugar, one tablespoonful of butter, eight tablespoonfuls of vinegar, one teaspoonful of salt and one of mustard. Mix the ingredients and steam in a double cooker until it is thick as ordinary cream. When ready to make the salad, the dressing should be thinned with cream or rich milk. If cream is used, whip it before adding the required amount of dressing. If put in a cool place, this dressing will keep for weeks and this amount is sufficient for several servings. —Mrs. E. A. Burnett.

SALAD DRESSING.

Three raw eggs, six tablespoonfuls of cream, three tablespoonfuls of sugar, three tablespoonfuls of melted butter, one teaspoonful of salt, one teaspoonful of mustard, a little pepper. Beat all together; add one cup of vinegar. Put on stove. Stir constantly until it thickens like custard, but do not let it boil.—Mrs. R. J. Walters.

SALMON SALAD.

Take a box of salmon, drain off all liquid and remove all pieces of skin and bone; break in pieces, not too small, then add a cup of chopped celery, a cup of chopped walnuts and three large apples chopped. Place in a dish and make a dressing of one cup of cream, butter size of a walnut, yolk of one egg, juice of one lemon, boil until it begins to thicken. When cold pour on mixture, then add one-half cup whipped cream.—Miss Geiken.

WALDORF SALAD.

Peel two raw apples and cut them into small pieces; also some celery and mix. Dress with a good mayonnaise. —Mrs. Noble.

CHICKEN SALMI.

Boil chicken or veal the day before and let broth jelly. The next morning put butter the size of an egg into stew-pan, when it bubbles throw in an even tablespoonful flour, cook thoroughly without browning. Mix into this a cupful a chicken broth, a cupful of boiling cream and one grating of nutmeg. At time chicken is boiled, put enough onion and celery in to season it. Cut up chicken in small pieces, add sweetbreads and mushrooms, one-third of each. Pour over this enough sauce to moisten as you would a rich salad dressing. Fill cups just as sent to table, putting a sprig of parsley in center of each. Do not allow to stand.

SALAD DRESSING.

Three eggs, one tablespoonful each of sugar and salt, two tablespoonfuls of oil, one (scant) of mustard, one cup of milk, in which is stirred a quarter teaspoonful of corn starch, one cup of vinegar. Stir oil, salt, sugar and mustard in a bowl until perfectly smooth. Add the egg well beaten, then vinegar and finally the milk. Put in the double boiler and stir while boiling until the dressing thickens like soft custard. Put in cold place and it will keep two weeks.—Mary E. Clarke.

SALAD DRESSING.

Six eggs, one-half cup sugar, one teaspoonful salt, one teaspoonful mustard, one teaspoonful flour, one-half cup butter, one cup vinegar, a little red pepper. Stir all together, cook in double boiler. When ready to use take out what you need and thin with whipped cream. For a fruit dressing add a little juice from the fruit.—Mrs. LeFevre.

SALAD DRESSING.

The yolks of five eggs well beaten, five tablespoons of vinegar, butter size of an egg, juice of half a lemon, one heaping tablespoonful of salad seasoning. Put vinegar into double boiler until it is boiling hot; add butter and stir in yolks slowly; when cool add lemon juice and seasoning and half a pint of heavy whipped cream.

To make seasoning: Six teaspoons of salt, four teaspoons of mustard one-half teaspoon of red pepper. Sift ten times.—Miss L. P. Averill.

SALAD DRESSING.

The yolks of four eggs, two-thirds of a cup of olive oil, red pepper, salt and mustard to taste; the juice of two lemons, and, last of all, one cup of thick cream. Be sure and put the cream in last, just before sending to the table.—Mrs. F. J. Meech.

VEGETABLES.

SCALLOPED POTATO.

Put into baking dish which has been greased, a layer of cold boiled potato, sliced thin; season with pepper and salt, also small pieces of butter; then layer of cracker crumbs. Season each layer; pour over a cup of sweet cream or chicken gravy; and bake.—Mrs. F. Butler.

FRIED TOMATOES (Maryland Style).

Take firm, ripe tomatoes, cut in halves, sprinkle with salt and pepper. Place them, cut side down, in a very hot frying pan in which have some bacon fat or lard; let them fry until brown; then turn, and when done, place in hot meat platter. Leave a few pieces in pan that have become broken and to these add salt, pepper and a generous lump of butter and enough cream to make plenty of gravy to fill the dish. Let the gravy boil up well.—Cora Lea Bentley.

SPAGHETTI.

One-half package broken, add one teaspoonful salt and quart boiling water. Let boil half hour, then drain. Fry one onion in butter until brown. Add one-half can tomatoes, spaghetti, one can mushrooms, one teaspoonful tabasco sauce and Worcestershire, a dash of red pepper. Put in baking dish and sprinkle grated cheese over and brown in oven.—Mrs. Chaloupka.

NOODLES—FRIED.

Two eggs beaten, and flour enough to roll. Dry and cut in three-inch squares and fry a minute in deep fat.—Mrs. Chaloupka.

SUCCOTASH.

Cook a cupful of Lima beans in salted water until almost done, then add the corn cut from five ears of tender sweet corn. Cook fifteen minutes, stirring constantly. The water should nearly all have cooked away by this time. Now add a little pepper, a chunk of butter about the size of a walnut and a cup of thin cream. Let boil up and serve. The beans should not be cooked too much or until they are mushy.—Mrs. Fred W. Mayne.

MACARONI CROQUETTES.

Cut fine one cupful cold macaroni; add this to a thick sauce made of one tablespoonful each of butter and flour and one cup of milk, tablespoonful of grated cheese, yolks of two eggs, salt, pepper. Cool, shape into balls and fry in deep fat.—Mrs. J. W. Harris.

VERMICELLI.

One-half pound vermicelli, one-fourth pound cream cheese, one pint tomatoes, one-half cup crackers or bread crumbs, two ounces butter, one-half pint milk, one teaspoonful Worcester sauce, salt and pepper. Boil vermicelli in plenty of water for fifteen or twenty minutes, until tender. Boil tomatoes three minutes by themselves, then skim vermicelli from water and place with tomatoes; let both cook five minutes, then add grated cheese, crumbs, sauce, salt and pepper to taste; lastly milk and butter. Let all come to boiling point and serve at once on toast or salted wafers. Will serve six persons.—Mrs. R. B. Armstrong.

SCALLOPED POTATOES.

Slice cold boiled potatoes and put layer in baking dish. Season with salt, pepper and butter and sprinkle with flour. Add another layer and so on until dish is about two-thirds full. Pour on milk nearly to the top of potato. Cover, and bake one hour, then remove cover and brown.—Mrs. P. A. Steed.

BOSTON BAKED BEANS.

Two and one-half pounds of beans, soak over night; in the morning parboil and about five minutes before draining add one-fourth of a teaspoon of soda; then put into bean pot, add one-half cup of sugar, three tablespoonfuls of molasses, one teaspoonful salt, two-thirds of a teaspoon black pepper, one pound of salt pork; fill pot with hot water; cover and bake several hours, occasionally adding water, so they do not become dry.—Mrs. J. Timmer.

POTATO PUFF.

Mould warm mashed cream potatoes in balls the size of a walnut; place in buttered tins and brush with well beaten egg. Set in a hot oven until brown. Serve hot.—Mrs. Tillotson.

Potatoes for baking will be much nicer if boiled ten or fifteen minutes before putting in oven to bake.—Mrs. E. E. Tillotson.

SCALLOPED CORN.

One can sweet corn, one pint of sweet milk, eight crackers rolled fine; season to taste. This should be put into baking dish in layers alternately. If corn is tender, bake twenty minutes.—Esther Van Alsburg.

MACARONI.

Macaroni should be broken and thoroughly washed in cold water and put into rapidly boiling salted water. Let it boil for thirty minutes, drain and plunge into cold water, where let it remain for about half an hour Drain and it is ready for the final cooking.—Mrs. R. W. Paddock.

MACARONI AND TOMATOES.

One-half pound macaroni, one-half can tomatoes, one tablespoonful of butter, one tablespoonful of flour. Season to taste. Boil macaroni as directed above. Put the butter in a frying pan; add a tablespoonful of flour. When mixed and brown add the tomatoes. Stir about ten minutes, then add the macaroni. When it boils it is ready to serve.—Mrs. R. W. Paddock.

POTATO CROQUETTES.

Season cold mashed potatoes with pepper, salt and nutmeg. Add a tablespoonful of butter to each pint of potato and then beat to a cream. Bind with two or three beaten eggs; add some minced parsley. Roll into oval balls, dip in beaten eggs, then in bread crumbs and fry in hot lard or drippings.—Mrs. B. Hartsig.

ITALIAN MACARONI.

(By an Italian Chef.)

One pound fresh link sausage, one quart can of tomatoes, two ordinary sized onions. Peel and slice onions and put all together to cook in granite basin on the back part of the stove. Cook slowly six to eight hours, being careful it does not burn. Remove the sausages (which are very nice boiled up in clear water for breakfast next morning). Boil a little less than one pound of macaroni broken in one-inch pieces, in salted water till tender. Grate or chop one pound cheese. In a large granite basin put a layer of the macaroni, a layer of cheese, salt and pepper to taste; then a layer of the tomatoes, enough to fill in crevices. Repeat these layers till the dish is full, sprinkling a layer of cheese on top. Bake in the oven fifteen or twenty minutes till nicely browned and serve hot.—Mrs. F. N. Chapel.

BAKED BEANS WITH TOMATOES.

Soak one quart of beans in cold water over night, put them on to cook in the morning, covering with fresh cold water and putting in one teaspoon soda. Boil until skins begin to crack. Then drain thoroughly, cover with boiling water. Take one-half pound salt pork, scrape and wash, cut off rind, slash across top one-half inch wide and one-half inch deep strips and sink it in beans. Add one pint cooked tomatoes, two tablespoons brown sugar or molasses. More salt if needed. Cook slowly until beans begin to break skin, then put in jar with meat, showing the cut top. Sprinkle with a very little sugar, to help them to brown. Pepper if liked.—Mrs. E. R. Sly, Bay Shore.

BREADS.

Sing a song of white bread,
Of brown bread and rye,
Find the kind that suits your taste,
Or tell the reason why.

YEAST BREAD.

When boiling potatoes for dinner take four medium-sized potatoes (well done) and mash fine. Add a little hot water and beat to a cream. Then add one tablespoonful of sugar, two cups of sifted flour and the water that the potatoes were boiled in, stirring constantly to beat out the lumps. When cool, add one cake of yeast foam, dissolved in lukewarm water, and put in a warm place to rise. Be careful not to scald.

The next morning sift three quarts of flour in a bread pan. Make a well in the center. Add one pint of lukewarm water to the yeast, two tablespoonfuls of salt and one tablespoonful of melted butter. Mix about as stiff as biscuit dough. Let rise until very light. Form in six loaves with only flour enough to shape the loaves. Do not get the dough too stiff, as that is what makes dry bread. Grease the top of the loaves with melted lard and let rise. Just before putting in the oven, prick the top of the loaves with a fork in three places, to let gas escape. Bake three-fourths of an hour in a good oven.—Mrs. Hattie J. Cooper.

GRAHAM LOAF.

One quart of Graham flour, two teaspoons Royal baking powder, one teaspoon of salt, one cup of brown sugar, milk enough to make batter, not too thick. Bake in a slow oven about half an hour.—Mrs. C. L. Gonser.

STEAMED BROWN BREAD.

Two cups of Graham flour, two cups of corn meal, one cup of molasses, three cups of sour milk, three teaspoonfuls of soda, one teaspoonful of salt. This makes five loaves in one-pound cans. Steam two hours.—Mrs. W. H. Woodley.

BROWN BREAD.

One and one-half cups sour milk, one-half cup molasses, one-half cup sugar, two cups Graham flour and one of white, one teaspoon soda, salt.—Mrs. Partridge.

STEAMED GRAHAM BREAD.

One cup sweet milk, one cup sour milk, one cup molasses, one teaspoonful Royal baking powder, one teaspoon soda. Stir all stiff with Graham flour. Steam two and one-half hours. Bake one-half hour.—Mrs. F. H. Hubbard.

GRAHAM BREAD.

One cup sour milk, one cup sweet milk, one-half cup molasses, a pinch of salt, a good teaspoon soda, one cup corn meal and two cups Graham flour. Bake one hour in an oven suitable for bread.—Mrs. J. A. Auld.

STEAMED BROWN BREAD.

One-half cup of sugar, one-half cup of molasses (scant), one-half teaspoonful soda put in the molasses, two cups of sweet milk, one cup of white flour, two cups of Graham flour, one teaspoonful baking powder, mixed in the flour. Steam two hours and bake one-half hour.—Mrs. J. E. Van Alsburg.

GRAHAM BREAD.

Two cups sour milk, one cup molasses (black strap or New Orleans), two teaspoons soda, three heaping cups Graham flour, butter size of egg, one-half teaspoon salt. Put in greased round tomato tin and steam two and one-half hours, then bake fifteen minutes, or bake in a slow oven one hour.—Mrs. F. E. Frazier.

BROWN BREAD.

Four cups of Graham flour, one cup of white flour, two teaspoonfuls of baking powder, one teaspoonful of salt, one cup of brown sugar or one-half cup of molasses. Add milk or milk and water to make a batter. (If sour milk is used, add soda.) Bake in a slow oven.—Mrs. R. B. Armstrong.

STEAMED BROWN BREAD.

One pint of sour milk or buttermilk, one-half teacup of molasses, pinch of salt, one pint of Indian meal, one pint of Graham flour, two teaspoons of soda dissolved in a tablespoon of water, one teacup of raisins or dates mixed in the flour. Steam one and one-half hours and bake fifteen minutes.—Mrs. H. P. Parmelee.

BROWN BREAD.

One cup corn meal, two cups grain flour, one cup sweet milk, one cup molasses, one cup sour milk, one teaspoonful soda, one teaspoonful salt. Steam three hours, then bake twenty minutes.—Mrs. Wm. Scroggie.

BOSTON BROWN BREAD.

One-half cup sugar, one and one-half cup molasses, one and one-half cups sour milk, one-third cup raisins, one teaspoon soda dissolved in hot water, one cup flour, one cup corn meal, one and one-half cups Graham flour. Steam two and one-half hours; bake fifteen minutes. Put on to steam over cold water, which is afterwards brought to boiling point and kept boiling.—Mrs. F. E. Frazier.

RYE BREAD.

Make yeast as for wheat bread, only have it a day older; the day before making your bread make a sponge with yeast and rye flour; the next morning set bread as for wheat bread by adding the desired warm water to sponge, then make the same as for wheat bread, only add shortening.—Mrs. G. L. Geiken.

CORN BREAD.

One cup of Indian meal, one cup of flour, one-half cup of sugar, one egg, one tablespoon of butter, one cup of sweet milk, a little salt, two teaspoons of baking powder.—Mrs. D. F. Meech.

GRAHAM BREAD.

One cup of molasses, two cups of sour milk or buttermilk, two cups of wheat flour, three cups of Graham flour, one small teaspoon of soda, raisins if desired, salt.—Mrs. D. F. Meech.

CORN BREAD.

One egg, one tablespoon sugar, one and one-half cups of sour cream, two tablespoonfuls of butter. If sour milk is used in place of cream, one teaspoonful of soda, a pinch of salt, one cup of flour and one cup of corn meal.—Mrs. W. H. Woodley.

JOHNNY CAKE.

One cup flour, two cups corn meal, one teaspoon salt, one tablespoon butter or drippngs, two tablespoons brown sugar, one teaspoon soda, one teaspoon cream of tartar, one egg, one cup of sour milk, more or less. Sweet milk may be used with one-half teaspoon soda, one teaspoon cream of tartar.—Mary E. Heston.

CORN BREAD.

One quart sweet milk boiled, stir in four tablespoonfuls corn meal; stand till cool; put in four beaten eggs, sweeten to taste; two tablespoonfuls butter. Bake two hours. Excellent.—Mrs. Finucan.

CORN BREAD.

Two cups sour milk, one-half cup sugar, two cups corn meal, one cup flour, piece of butter size of walnut, two small teaspoons of soda, one stiffly beaten egg, the white added last. Bake thirty minutes.—Mrs. Owen M. Wood.

SPOON CORN BREAD (Virginia Recipe).

One pint sour milk, one egg, two large iron spoonfuls corn meal, one-half teaspoon soda, a little salt. Mix and bake in square tins.—Mrs. Gears.

JOHNNY CAKE.

One tablespoon of butter, one cup of sugar, two eggs, one cup flour, one cup sour cream, one teaspoon soda, one cup corn meal Beat eggs, butter and sugar together; add cream (or rich buttermilk, then meal and flour.—Miss Dorothy Iddings.

CORN DODGERS.

Scald one quart corn meal with one or more cups of boiling water. Add one tablespoonful of melted lard and one teaspoonful of salt, also enough hot water to make a soft dough. Mold by the handful into an oval shape. Bake in quick oven.—Mrs. Wm. Scroggie.

JOHNNY CAKE.

One and one-half cups of sour milk, two tablespoons of sugar, one egg, one scant teaspoon soda, one cup of flour, two cups of corn meal, pinch of salt.—Mrs. Babcock.

BUNS.

When the bread dough is ready for the loaves, take enough dough for one loaf and add one-half cupful of shortening (half butter and half lard), and one-half cupful of sugar. Mix thoroughly, adding flour as necessary to work smooth. Let rise until very light, then roll out, cut into buns and let rise again. Bake about twenty minutes. Cover tops with a syrup made by boiling sugar and water while the buns bake.—Mrs. Auld.

ENGLISH BUNS.

Sift together one quart flour, two dessertspoons baking powder, rub in butter size of an egg, beat two eggs light, add one cup sugar, one pint milk and water mixed; stir into the mixture, roll out, cut in cakes, bake in hot oven. Add raisins or currants.—Mrs. Frank Payne.

PIES.

"Parvus Jacobus Horner,
Sedebat in a corner,
Edens a Christmas pie;
Inferuit thumb,—Extraherit plum—
Clamans—'Quid sharp puer am I'—."

TRANSPARENT PIE.

Line small tin patty pans with pie crust. Line the crusts with peach preserves. Beat the yolks of six eggs and the whites of two eggs to a froth. Cream one cup butter and two cups of sugar. Beat all together well. Flavor with nutmeg, pour over the peaches and bake. This makes twenty-four individual pies.—Mrs. B. W. Miller.

LEMON CREAM PIE.

The juice of one lemon, one cupful of sugar, yolks of two eggs, two tablespoonfuls of flour, mix all together and pour over one cupful boiling water. Cook in a double boiler until thick. Make a pie with an under crust only, and bake it; then put in the filling and spread over the pie a frosting made of the whites of two eggs and two tablespoonfuls sugar. Return to oven and brown slightly.—Mrs. J. E. Van Alsburg.

BANANA PIE.

Bake an under crust. While warm fill it with sliced bananas. Sprinkle over them pulverized sugar and the juice of one orange. Frost with whipped cream and serve. —Esther Van Alsburg.

CREAM PIE.

One-half pint of new milk, one-half cupful sugar, two tablespoonfuls corn starch, two eggs (yolks only), pinch of salt. Mix the corn starch with a little of the cold milk, add the sugar, salt and beaten eggs. Put the remainder of the milk on the stove, and when boiling hot stir in the other ingredients. Boil all together until it thickens. Have two pie crusts baked ready for the cream, and put in as soon as it is done. For frosting, beat the whites of the eggs stiff; add two tablespoonfuls of powdered sugar. Brown in oven two or three minutes.—Mrs. A. M. Burdick.

MINCE MEAT FOR PIES.

Three bowls of chopped meat, five of apples, four of sugar, one of New Orleans molasses, one of cider or not too strong vinegar. Two bowls of raisins or part currants, one of fruit syrup of a mixture of jellies, preserved cherries and any little left-overs; also add one small bowl of suet chopped very fine or a generous piece of butter, two tablespoonfuls cinnamon, two of cloves, one of salt, one or two nutmegs. Citron if you like.—Mrs. F. E. Wood.

CHESS CAKE.

One pound of sugar, half pound of butter, yolks of twelve eggs, whites of two, flavor with lemon. Cream the butter well. Beat the eggs until very light, then add the sugar and stir this slowly into the butter. After all is well mixed put into a rich pastry (in pie pans) and bake. When done, make the unused whites into a meringue and put over the top, then put back into the oven just long enough to brown lightly. Remove from stove and while hot cut into slices; this will prevent their falling.—Mrs. John C. New.

WASHINGTON PIE.

One cup sugar, one egg, one-half cup of milk, one cup flour, one teaspoonful baking powder. Stir and bake in two cake tins.

Filling.—Three full cups of milk, one egg, one-third cup of flour, one-half cup of sugar, pinch of salt. Put the milk to boil. Beat the other ingredients well together and stir into the boiling milk. When thick, add vanilla to flavor. When cold put between the layers as for jelly cake.—Mrs. O. D. Wood.

APPLE PIE (Clyde's Favorite).

Make rich crust with one cup lard, one tablespoonful salt, cut thoroughly into three cups flour. (This will make three pies.) Sprinkle corn starch on bottom crust (use corn starch same way for all fruit pies), cut apples in quarters, place on end round and round until the pie tin is full. Sprinkle on three-fourths cup brown sugar more or less, one-half teaspoon salt, one teaspoon allspice and grated nutmeg, some bits of butter, add three tablespoonfuls water, then sprinkle on corn starch, wet the edge of bottom crust, put on top crust with ornamental opening for steam escape and bake three-fourths of an hour or more.—Mrs. M. E. Heston.

ROLLED MEAT PIE.

One quart flour, two teaspoonfuls baking powder, one-half teaspoonful salt, one-half cup lard or butter. Use milk or water to make a soft dough and roll one-fourth inch thick.

Filling.—One-half pound beef, one-half pound pork, boil until tender, chop fine, season with salt, pepper, and onion if liked. Moisten with liquid from meat, spread on rolled crust. Roll up as jell cake and bake one-half hour in buttered tin in moderately heated oven. Put on platter and cover with liquid from meat thickened with flour and seasoned.—Mrs. M. W. LaPier.

MINCE MEAT.

Three pounds of meat, two pounds chopped suet, three and one-half pounds of apples, two and one-half pounds of raisins and currants, two cups of molasses, spices and sugar to taste; odds and ends of fruit may be added. Cider to thin.—Mrs. A. Ross.

MINCE MEAT.

Five bowls of chopped meat (which has been stewed), nine bowls of chopped apples, four bowls of sugar, one bowl of vinegar, one bowl molasses, one bowl of fruit juice, one bowl of cider, three pounds of raisins, two tablespoonfuls each of cinnamon and cloves, three nutmegs, one tablespoonful salt.—Mrs. H. Van Alsburg.

MOTHER'S ONE-CRUSTED APPLE PIE.

Fill a deep pie plate with very thinly sliced tart apples, sprinkled with sugar, nutmeg, and a little water. Cover with a thin piecrust and bake in quick oven. Remove the crust, turn upside down in a large dinner plate, leaving the apples in the pie plate. Mix well, adding more sugar, if necessary, and then place in the crust. Serve as soon as possible with cream.—Cora Lea Bentley.

CHOCOLATE PIE.

Cook a nice flaky shell and fill with the following: One-half cup of granulated sugar, to which add two tablespoonfuls of grated chocolate, one tablespoonful of flour. Mix and add the yolks of two eggs and one and one-half cups of milk. Put on the stove and cook until it thickens, stirring constantly. When cool spread over the top the whites of two eggs beaten to a stiff froth with a little sugar. Put in oven to brown.—Mrs. F. M. Harris.

PIE CRUST.

One cup of flour, two tablespoons lard, three tablespoons of water, a little salt.—Miss Stoudt.

MOCK CREAM PIE.

Make two pie crusts, and bake. For filling, one quart of milk put in a spider and boil. Yolks of three eggs and one white, one cup of sugar, one-half cup of flour. Mix and stir into the boiling milk, and boil until thick. One teaspoon of vanilla. Pour into the crusts, and frost with the whites.—Mrs. A. Wood.

AMBER PIE.

Three-fourths cup granulated sugar, one tablespoonful flour stirred in sugar, one large tablespoonful butter. Rub sugar and butter together. One-half cup sour cream, one-half cup blackberry jelly, or any kind convenient, four eggs, yolks only. Save the whites for meringue.—Mrs. John C. New.

PUDDINGS.

APPLE FROSTING FOR PUDDING SAUCE.

One cup sugar, two tablespoonfuls grated apple, white of one egg. Beat to a very stiff froth. Flavor with extract if desired.—Mrs. A. L. Coulter.

BAKED INDIAN PUDDING.

One quart sweet milk, one ounce butter (size of a small egg), one teacup corn meal, four well beaten eggs, one-half pound raisins, one-half cup sugar. Scald milk and stir in meal while boiling. Let stand till blood warm. Stir all well together. Bake one and one-half hours. Serve with sauce.

Sauce.—One cup sugar, one lemon (juice and rind), one tablespoonful corn starch, a little butter. Beat all together and just before serving add one-half pint boiling water. Fine.

SUET PUDDING.

One cup suet chopped fine, one cup molasses, one cup sweet milk, three and one-half cups flour, one cup raisins, one teaspoonful soda dissolved in a little boiling water. Steam two hours.

Sauce for Same.—One cup sugar, one-fourth cup butter, one egg, one tablespoonful vinegar, grated rind and juice of one lemon, three tablespoonfuls water. Beat well and bring to a boil. Serve hot. Very fine.—Mrs. G. C. Geiken.

FRUIT STEAMED PUDDING.

One pint of flour, heaping dessert spoon of baking powder. Milk enough to make batter so it will not run. Steam thirty minutes.

Sauce.—Cream one-half cup of butter, one cup of sugar. Add beaten white of an egg, two cups of crushed or canned berries. I prefer raspberries.—Mrs. Priest.

PRUNE PUDDING.

Stew one-half pound of prunes until tender with very little water, add one-half cup of sugar; when cold press through a sieve and add whites of six eggs well beaten. Set pudding dish in a pan of water and bake in slow oven for thirty or forty minutes. Serve cold with whipped cream.—Miss K. L. Meech.

GRAHAM PUDDING.

Two cups Graham flour, one cup seeded raisins, one-half cup molasses, two cups sweet milk with two small teaspoons soda stirred in milk, salt. Steam two hours and serve with sweet sauce.—Mrs. Frank Payne.

GRAHAM PUDDING.

One egg, one cup each of sweet milk, molasses (or for sweetening may be used one-half cup brown sugar and one-half cup molasses), Graham flour, white flour and fruit. Level teaspoon of soda. Steam two hours.

Sauce.—One scant half-cup butter, one cup powdered sugar. Cream butter and sugar together and add two well beaten eggs, drop by drop. Flavor. Stir all until it separates. For double, use thiee eggs. Fine.—Mrs. Nettie Priest.

SUET OR POOR MAN'S PUDDING.

One cup of suet, one-half cup of molasses, one cup of milk, one egg, one cup seeded raisins, two tablespoonfuls of sugar, two cups of flour with two teaspoonfuls baking powder. A little salt.—Mrs. Jean P. Crawford.

APPLE TAPIOCA PUDDING.

Put two-thirds cup of tapioca and a teaspoonful of salt into a pint of water and let stand two or three hours where it will be quite warm, but not cook. Peel, quarter and core enough tart apples to cover the bottom of a two-quart pudding dish. Add one-half cup sugar and a little nutmeg. Then add to the tapioca one cup milk, one-half cup sugar, a teaspoon of butter, not melted, and a little nutmeg, and pour over the apples. Let bake in a moderate oven about an hour. Be sure the apples are cooked. To be eaten warm with cream or any sweet pudding sauce.—Mrs. A. F. Bridge.

QUEEN OF PUDDINGS.

One and one-half pints of fine bread crumbs, add a small quart of milk, the yolks of four eggs beaten well, the grated peel of a lemon, a piece of butter the size of an egg, added in small pieces. Bake until done, but not watery. Spread over the pudding a layer of jelly or jam. Whip the whites of the four eggs to a stiff froth and beat in a teacup of sugar in which has been stirred the juice of the lemon. Pour whites over the jam and put in the oven to brown slightly. To be eaten cold with cream.—Miss K. L. Meech.

CHOCOLATE PUDDING.

One quart of milk scalded, one and one-half squares of chocolate grated, wet with cold milk and stirred into the scalded milk. When chocolate is dissolved, take two heaping tablespoonfuls corn starch, six tablespoonfuls sugar, yolks of three eggs well beaten. Cook until quite thick. Beat the whites of eggs stiff with sugar; then spread over the top. Left in oven until light brown.—Mrs. John A. Crawford.

COTTAGE PUDDING.

Two eggs, one small cup sugar, one-half cup melted butter, one-half cup sweet milk, salt and spice, two cups flour, two teaspoonfuls baking powder sifted with flour. Serve with sweet sauce.—Mrs. Frank Payne.

BUCKEYE PUDDING.

One cup of chopped raisins, one and one-half cups of molasses, one cup of warm water, two and one-half cups of flour, one dessert spoonful of soda, yolks of two eggs. Steam two hours.

Sauce.—One cup of sugar, one-half cup of butter, one teaspoonful warm water, cream. Add beaten whites of two eggs. Just before serving, flavor with lemon.—Mrs. H. D. Marshall.

CREAM PUFFS.

One-half cup butter, one cup water, one cup flour, three eggs. Melt butter in hot water. When it boils stir in flour. Take from fire and let cool, and when cold stir in three eggs, one at a time (without beating). Drop on buttered tins, bake in a hot oven twenty to thirty minutes. Open from side and fill.

Filling.—One egg, one cup sweet milk, one-half cup sugar, a little corn starch, vanilla flavoring. Cook in double boiler.—Mrs. L. E. Benton.

SNOW PUDDING.

One-half box of gelatine, one cup of sugar, one and one-half pints of water, three eggs, lemon flavoring, milk. Flavor the sugar and gelatine with lemon juice and put into the water and boil for a few minutes. When the jelly is quite cold and nearly set, put in the egg whites beaten stiff and beat all together for thirty minutes, or until it has the appearance of snow. Turn into a mold; serve very cold. Make a sauce of egg yolks and milk enough to make a thin custard.—Mrs. Bert Van Allsburg.

STEAMED MOLASSES PUDDING.

One cup of hot water, one cup of molasses, one tablespoonful melted butter, one teaspoonful soda. Flour until thick. Fruit or spices. Steam two hours. Serve with hot sauce.

NESSELRODE PUDDING.

Make a syrup of one and one-quarter cups of sugar and one-half cup of water; beat the yolks of six eggs until light; pour the syrup over them, beating all the time. Cook over hot water until it makes a thick coating on the spoon; remove from the fire and beat until cold. Pour in one quart of cream; freeze until it begins to thicken; put into it one-quarter pound of candied fruits cut in pieces, one cup of almonds blanched and pounded. Continue to freeze until stiff. This pudding can be made richer by adding one cup of seeded raisins cut in pieces and one-half can of grated pineapple.—Mrs. D. F. Meech.

STEAMED FIG PUDDING.

One cup of chopped suet, one and one-half cups of chopped bread crumbs, one cup of sugar, three-fourths pounds of figs chopped fine, four eggs, one cup of milk, one nutmeg, one and one-half teaspoons of baking powder. Steam three hours. Serve with any sweet pudding sauce. —Nelle Burnett Hinchey.

CHERRY PUDDING.

One cup sugar, two tablespoonfuls melted butter, two eggs, one cup milk, two cups flour, two teaspoonfuls baking powder. Put preserved cherries in bottom of buttered pudding dish, pour the mixture on top and steam three-quarters of an hour. Turn pudding out on a dish, leaving fruit on top. For the sauce, cream one cup sugar, one-half cup butter, add one cupful of cherry juice, heated.—Mrs. Herschell Miller.

A FAVORITE PUDDING.

One cup flour, one-half cup sugar, two eggs, one tablespoonful butter, one tablespoonful milk, one teaspoonful soda, one tablespoonful jelly. Cream the butter and sugar; add jelly, then yolks of eggs, then flour, a pinch of salt, and soda dissolved in the milk, then the whites beaten to a stiff froth and last a little flavoring. Butter a dish, pour in the mixture, cover with buttered paper and steam one hour. Serve with any sauce preferred.—Mrs. C. E. Miller.

STEAMED GRAHAM PUDDING.

One cup sour milk, one cup molasses, one cup raisins, two and one-half cups Graham flour, two level teaspoonfuls soda, pinch of salt. Steam two hours.

Sauce for above.—One cup sugar, one cup boiling water, butter size of a walnut, one tablespoonful vinegar, one teaspoonful lemon extract, nutmeg. Let come to a boil and thicken with a little flour or corn starch.—Mrs. J. A. Auld.

HOSPITAL PUDDING.

One cup molasses, one cup hot water, one egg, salt. Dissolve one teaspoonful soda in water. Flour thick enough to lap. Steam two hours.

Sauce.—Cream butter and sugar and gradually add hot milk. Season with vanilla.—Mrs. George Smith.

CREAMY SAUCE.

Beat a half cupful butter to a cream, and stir in a half cupful of powdered sugar. When very light, add three tablespoonfuls of cream, a little at a time. Put the dish in a pan of boiling water, and stir until the sauce is very smooth and creamy, but not longer. Add flavoring, and serve.—Mrs. Herschell Miller.

FRUIT PUDDING.

Three cups bread crumbs, one-half cup butter, one cup entire wheat flour, one-half teaspoonful salt, one teaspoon cinnamon, one-half nutmeg, one teaspoonful soda, one-half teaspoonful baking powder, three-fourths cup molasses, two apples chopped fine, one cup raisins, one cup currants, two cups milk. Mix crumbs and butter with finger tips, then add flour, then remainder of ingredients. Steam for three hours. Serve with following sauce:

Four tablespoonfuls butter, gradually add one cup powdered sugar, beat to a cream, then add the stiffly beaten white of one egg, flavor with lemon or vanilla.—Mrs. B. Hartsig.

LEMON PUDDING.

The yolk of four eggs and four tablespoonfuls sugar, juice and rind of one lemon, butter the size of a walnut. Mix thoroughly, put in Farina boiler and stir until it thickens. Whites of the four eggs beaten and stirred in the last thing. White of one egg beaten stiff, add tablespoon heaping full sugar and frost over top of pudding.—Hattie A. Brown.

BAKED LEMON PUDDING.

Heat one pint sweet milk and pour over one cup of bread crumbs; add a small piece of butter and let this stand until cool. When cool, add the well beaten yolks of two eggs, one-half cup sugar and the grated rind of one lemon. Bake in a buttered dish until firm and slightly brown, from a half to three-quarters of an hour. When done cover with a meringue made of the well beaten whites of two eggs, four tablespoonfuls sugar and the juice of one lemon. Put back in oven and brown.—Mrs. H. R. Fowler.

CREAM PUFFS.

Stew one-half pound prunes, when cold remove the stone, and chop fine, beat the whites of three eggs stiff, add six tablespoons of sugar, and beat in the chopped prunes, whip hard for three minutes, and turn into a greased pudding dish, bake in a hot oven for half an hour, serve immediately with whipped cream.—Mrs. J. B. Parsons.

ESTELLE PUDDING.

Three well beaten eggs, two and one-half tablespoonfuls of sugar, two tablespoonfuls of butter, three-fourths of a cup of sweet milk, one cup of chopped raisins, cranberries, figs or dates, one even tablespoonful of baking powder sifted into flour enough to make like cake batter. Steam thirty-five minutes in molds. Excellent with figs and dates, served with whipped cream, sweetened and flavored.—Mrs. E. V. Madison.

RAISIN PUFFS.

One-half cup of butter, one cup of sugar, two eggs, one cnp of sweet milk, two cups of flour, two teaspoonfuls Royal baking powder, one cup of raisins. Put into cups and steam one and one-half hours. Serve with sauce.

Sauce.—One cup of boiling water, two tablespoonfuls corn starch, four tablespoonfuls vinegar, two tablespoonfuls of butter, one and a half cups of sugar. Flavor to suit the taste.—Mrs. J. E. Van Alsburg.

LEMON PUDDING.

Two and one-half cups boiling water, juice of one lemon, one cup sugar and two tablespoonfuls corn starch. Cook until clear and when cool add the well beaten whites of three eggs and pour into moulds. Serve with custard sauce.

Custard Sauce.—Beat yolks of three eggs and one cup granulated sugar, add to one pint warm milk and cook until it begins to thicken, stirring constantly.—Mrs. F. E. Cartier.

STEAMED FRUIT PUDDING.

One tablespoonful sugar, one egg, piece of butter size of an egg. Stir to a cream. Sift in one pint flour, two tablespoonfuls baking powder and sufficient milk or water to make drop batter. Butter six pudding cups, put one spoonful batter in each and then a tablespoon of berries or fruit free from syrup, then another spoonful batter. Steam thirty minutes.

Sauce for above.—One cup fruit, three-fourths cup sugar, one and one-half cups hot water. Put sugar and berries together, add the water, place in double boiler with piece of butter size of an egg. Thicken with one tablespoonful corn starch dissolved in a little water, cook until clear.—Mrs. L. E. Benton.

APPLE DUMPLINGS.

Make as for biscuit, only richer, a baking powder crust, Roll to a half-inch in thickness and cut out as for biscuit. Peel and quarter some good tart apples; fill the dough with apples, a little piece of butter; press the edges firmly together. Put into a deep baking dish a scant cup sugar, a piece of butter size of a large egg. Season with nutmeg or cinnamon and pour on boiling water until the dumplings are all covered but the top. Bake forty or fifty minutes. Serve with cream and sugar or any good sauce, and put on each some of the syrup they are baked in.—Mrs. Edyth E. Stacks.

SUET PUDDING (Fine).

One cup chopped suet, one cup chopped raisins, one cup New Orleans molasses, teaspoon each of ground cloves, cinnamon, salt, soda, one cup sweet milk, three and one-half cups flour more or less. Steam three hours.

Sauce.—One-half cup butter, one cup sugar, one tablespoon flour, creamed, one cup boiling water. Boil until smooth (two minutes), flavor with lemon.—Mary E. Heston.

DELICIOUS BREAD PUDDING.

One-half pint bread crumbs, one pint sweet milk, yolks of two eggs, one-half cup sugar, grated lemon rind, butter size small egg. Turn in pudding dish, put in a pan of water and bake till it thickens, about one-half hour. Take out and squeeze over it the juice of a lemon. Cover with beaten whites, sweten and brown. Serve hot.—Mrs. George Smith.

SNOW PUDDING.

Whites of two eggs, two tablespoonfuls gelatine soaked in cold water two hours, then dissolve it with boiling water. Add to the dissolved gelatine one-half cup granulated sugar. Flavor with vanilla. When this mixture is cold, add it to the well beaten whites. Then beat the whole thoroughly. Add chopped nuts and chopped candied fruits if desired. Put in a mold to harden. Serve with custard sauce.—Mrs. Fred Smith.

OATMEAL PUDDING.

One cup cooked oatmeal, two eggs, one-fourth cup sugar, one teaspoonful lemon extract, one-half cup raisins, one quart sweet milk.—Mrs. C. E. See.

PUDDING.

Make orange jelly. Put it into a mould, put a smaller mould or bowl in the center of this that will leave a hole when the jelly is in form. When jelly is in form whip one pint of thick cream, flavor with vanilla, into which stir two tablespoonfuls thoroughly cooked rice which should be in kernels, one-half cup sugar, and about two heaping spoonfuls cut-up candied fruit and chopped nuts if you like. Stir all together and fill in the hole in the jelly with the prepared rice and whipped cream. Let stand for two hours before turning out to serve. Put whipped cream around the form of jelly.—Mrs. Fred Smith.

BAKED CHOCOLATE CUSTARDS.

For five small custards use one pint of milk, two eggs, one ounce of chocolate, one-quarter of a teaspoonful of salt, and a piece of stick cinnamon about an inch long. Put the cinnamon and milk in the double boiler, place on the fire and cook for ten minutes. Shave the chocolate and put it in a small pan with three tablespoonfuls of sugar and one of boiling water. Stir this over a hot fire until smooth and glossy and then stir it into the hot milk, after which take the liquid mixture from the fire and cool. Beat together with a spoon the eggs, salt and two tablespoonfuls of the sugar. Add the cooled milk and strain. Pour the mixture into the cups which place in a deep pan. Pour into the pan enough tepid water to come nearly to the top of the cups. Place in the oven to bake. It will take about half an hour. Test by running a knife through the center. If the custard is milky it is not done. Serve cold.—Mrs. Sears, Oak Park, Ill.

SUET PUDDING.

One cup chopped suet, one cup chopped raisins, one cup sour milk, one teaspoonful cinnamon, one-half teaspoonful allspice, one-half cup molasses, two eggs, one teaspoonful soda (heaping). Stir very thick.—Mrs. Arthur L. Fitch.

CORN STARCH PUDDING.

One pint sweet milk, whites of three eggs, two tablespoonfuls corn starch, three of sugar. Put the milk into a double boiler and when it reaches the boiling point add the sugar, then the starch dissolved in a little cold milk, and lastly the whites of eggs whipped to a stiff froth; beat and let stand a few minutes, then pour into moulds.

Sauce.—One pint milk, three tablespoonfuls sugar and yolks well beaten. Flavor with vanilla.—Lillian Compton.

PINEAPPLE TAPIOCA.

One cup tapioca, one cup sugar, one can grated pineapple. Soak tapioca, boil in water until done, add sugar, then pineapple. Serve when cold with cream.—Edna Sue Green.

SUET PUDDING.

Mix one cup of stoned raisins, one cup of currants, one cup of chopped suet, one-half teaspoonful of cinnamon, one-half grated nutmeg, with three and one-half cups of dried bread crumbs, one cup of molasses, one cup of sweet milk, a good pinch of salt, one teaspoonful of soda in a spoon of milk; mix dry and wet ingredients together with one well beaten egg. Pour into a two-quart pan and steam three hours. Serve with lemon sauce or whipped cream.—Genevieve Jarvis.

LEMON PUDDING.

Two eggs, the yolks, one-half cup sugar, one pint of milk, one-half pint of bread crumbs, one-half teaspoonful of butter, the grated rind of one lemon. When well done spread over the top a layer of jelly and add the whites of the eggs whipped to a stiff froth, sweetened with one cup of sugar and flavored with juice of lemon. Set in oven to brown slightly. Allow half an hour for baking.—Genevieve Jarvis.

GRAHAM PUDDING.

One and one-half cups molasses, one-half cup sweet milk, one of fruit, two eggs, one tablespoonful butter, one teaspoonful of soda, one and one-half cups of Graham flour. Steam one and one-half hours.—Mrs. F. E. Wood.

CHOCOLATE BREAD PUDDING.

Ten tablespoonfuls of grated bread, five tablespoonfuls of grated (unsweetened) chocolate, one quart of sweet milk, pinch of salt. Put into double boiler and scald. Remove from stove, add one cup of sugar (which will cool the milk), one teaspoonful of vanilla, yolks of three eggs well beaten. Bake in moderate oven. When baked use the whites of three eggs for frosting, adding one tablespoonful sugar. Spread over pudding, return to oven and brown. Serve with sweet cream, or any sauce desired. When baking the pudding test with a knife. Very good.—Mrs. W. E. Bedwin.

PUFF PUDDING.

One pint flour, two teaspoonfuls baking powder, the well beaten white of one egg, add milk to make of the consistency of white cake. Grease some cups, put in one tablespoonful of the mixture and a tablespoonful of fruit, cover with another tablespoonful of the mixture. Steam three-fourths of an hour and serve with any liquid sauce.—Mrs. H. R. Fowler.

ENGLISH PUDDING.

One and one-half cups suet, one and one-half cups sugar, one cup bread crumbs, two cups flour, one cup water, three eggs, two teaspoonfuls cinnamon, one teaspoonful cloves, one-half teaspoonful nutmeg, two cups raisins, two cups currants. Steam three hours. May be eaten with any sauce.—Mrs. Grace Hyres.

PLUM PUDDING.

One-half pound brown sugar, one-half pound suet chopped fine, three eggs, one-half pint sweet milk, one-half pound raisins, also same of currants if so desired, one teaspoonful of soda, spice to taste, and flour to make a very stiff batter. Steam three hours. Whipped cream is delicious with the above, or one may use any desired sauce.—Mrs. Edith Vickers.

STEAMED PUDDING.

One egg, two tablespoonfuls of sugar, two tablespoonfuls of butter, one-half cup of molasses, one and one-half cups of sifted flour, one teaspoonful of soda, one-half cup of boiling water. Steam one hour.

Sauce.—Cream together two egg yolks and one cup of granulated sugar. Add one cup of whipped cream. Flavor with vanilla.—Mary Dunham Shanahan.

BAKED INDIAN PUDDING.

One quart sweet milk, butter size of an egg, one teacup corn meal, four well beaten eggs, one-half pound raisins, one-half cup sugar. Scald milk and stir in meal while boiling. Let stand until lukewarm, then stir all together thoroughly.

Sauce.—One cup sugar, one lemon, juice and rind, one tablespoonful corn starch, butter size of a walnut. Beat sugar, lemon and butter together. Boil the corn starch in enough water to make one-half pint when cooked. Add this to the other ingredients just before serving.—Mrs. T. F. Thomas.

ANGEL FOOD PUDDING.

Chop together one cup English walnut meats, and one cup of stoned dates. Add one small cup sugar, two tablespoonfuls of flour and one teaspoonful baking powder. Bake in a buttered dish in moderate oven for twenty minutes. Serve with cream, whipped or plain. This is sufficient quantity to serve four people.—Mrs. A. T. Burnett.

PRUNE PUDDING.

Wash and remove stones from one pound of good prunes. Soak over night in plenty of water. When the dessert is to be prepared drain the prunes well and chop fine, then add one-half cup of sugar, one teaspoon of vanilla, and two well beaten eggs and stir thoroughly. Chill and serve with cream. Chopped English walnut meats may be added to this pudding if desired. One-half cupful is a good proportion. Do not attempt to cook the prunes as the pudding has a finer flavor if they are uncooked.—Mrs. E. A. Burnett.

BLACK HAWK CLUB PUDDING.

Beat two eggs, one-half cup sugar, and one-half teaspoon salt. Add one-half cup molasses, one-half cup sour cream, one-half teaspoon soda, a few raisins and flour to make a stiff batter. Steam one and one-half hours. Serve with liquid, hot sauce.—Mrs. R. W. Paddock.

YORKSHIRE PUDDING.

To be eaten wth roast beef. Two cups flour, stir in two teaspoons of baking powder, half teaspoon salt, add slowly one quart milk, stir in three beaten eggs; pour around roast half hour before meat is done.—Mrs. J. B. Thielen.

PINEAPPLE TAPIOCA PUDDING.

Soak one-third cup of pearl tapioca over night. In the morning cook until clear after adding to it one-half cup of water, one-half cup of sugar and one-half cup of pineapple chopped fine; beat white of one egg very stiff and add the juice of half a lemon, pour this slowly into the cooked mixture, beating all the time; continue beating fifteen minutes or until light. Serve with whipped cream sweetened, or jelly, or with hot sweetened chocolate.—Mrs. Fred W. Mayne.

APPLE DUMPLINGS.

One-half cup lard, one quart flour, two teaspoonfuls baking powder, salt, milk enough to roll out, cut in squares, fill center with apples cut in quarters, sprinkle with sugar and cinnamon, cut butter in small pieces and place on top. Pinch dough together, brush with cold water, bake forty minutes; ten minutes before done brush tops with yolk of one egg beaten with one tablespoonful sugar to glaze them, serve with the following sauce: Take four tart apples, pare and grate, sprinkle with sugar, break white of two eggs into apples beat twenty minutes.—Mrs. John Ackart, Jr.

Make cup custard in cups and serve with maple syrup.

CHOCOLATE PUFFS.

One-half cup of sugar, one tablespoon of butter, one egg, two squares of Baker's chocolate grated, one-half cup of milk, one cup of flour, one teaspoon of Royal baking powder; steam one hour. This makes five or six puffs in good-sized patty pans, or small teacups may be used in the steamer. To be served hot with sugar and cream, or the following sauce may be used:

Sauce.—Yolks of two eggs, one cup of powdered sugar, beaten together; flavor with vanilla; add one-half pint of whipped cream; if too thick a little unbeaten cream can be added.—O. A. Sears.

CHAUTAUQUA PUDDING.

Three-fourths of a cup of maple syrup, one cupful milk, one cupful raisins, one teaspoonful soda, one-half teaspoonful salt, butter size of an egg, flour to make stiff as cake batter. Steam three hours.

Sauce.—Six tablespoonfuls of sugar, four tablespoonfuls of butter, two tablespoonfuls of flour, stir to a cream, then add boiling water. Boil until it thickens, flavor with vanilla.—Mrs. John Ackert, Jr.

BAKED LEMON PUDDING.

One quart milk, two cups of bread crumbs, four eggs, whites and yolks beaten separately, one tablespoonful butter, one cup of white sugar, one lemon, juice and grated rind. Heat the milk and pour over the bread crumbs; add the butter, cover and let get soft; when cool beat the sugar and yolks and add the grated rind. Bake in buttered dish until firm and slightly brown, from one-half to three-fourths of an hour. When done cover with the whites of eggs whipped to a stiff froth with four tablespoonfuls of powdered sugar and the lemon juice. Return to the oven and brown.

Lemon Sauce for Same.—One cup sugar, one-half cup butter, one egg beaten light, one lemon, juice and grated rind, one-half cup boiling water. Pour in granite basin and thicken over steam.—Mrs. Hattie J. Cooper.

CARROT PUDDING.

Three-fourths cup of flour, one-half cup sugar, one-half cup suet, one-half cup raisins, one-half cup raw potatoes (grated), two and one-half cups raw carrots (grated), one small teaspoon soda. Steam two and one-half hours.—Mrs. Frank Sears.

SUET PUDDING.

One cup of chopped fruit (raisins or currants), one cup of chopped suet, one-half cup molasses, one-half cup dark sugar, one teaspoonful of soda, two teacups sweet milk, one-half teaspoon salt. Steam three hours.

Sauce.—One cup sugar, one-half cup butter, yolks of two eggs, one wine-glass vinegar. Rub butter and sugar together until creamy, add eggs and half the vinegar. Put the dish in boiling water and stir ten minutes and add the rest of the vinegar. This pudding will keep nicely and can be steamed over when wanted.—Mrs. C. L. Gonser.

CARROT PUDDING.

One cup chopped suet, one cup sugar, one cup raisins, one cup currants, one cup grated potato, one cup grated carrot, one and one-half cups flour, three-quarters teaspoonful soda dissolved in warm water, salt. Knead into loaf and steam three hours. Can put in more fruit if desired.—Mrs. Lamoreaux.

ICES and DESSERTS.

CHARLOTTE RUSSE.

Four eggs, one ounce gelatine, one teacup sugar, one pint of milk, one pint of cream; beat thoroughly the yolks with the sugar, the whites separately. Dissolve the gelatine in the pint of milk, season with vanilla; add the ingredients, beating them well. Whip the cream to a froth and add to the mixture. Line two moulds with sponge cake and pour the mixture over it. Set in a cool place until congealed.—Mrs. O. D. Wood.

Bananas dipped in beaten egg, then rolled in chopped walnut meats and placed in a pan in the oven for a few minutes make an appetizing dessert.

PRUNE WHIP.

Take one pound best prunes, wash thoroughly and leave in water over night; then stew slowly until soft. While hot remove the pits, add one-half cup granulated sugar, boil until the syrup is well cooked into the prunes. Beat the whites of six eggs to a light froth, add one teacup of pulverized sugar and again beat rapidly for fifteen minutes. Turn the frosting upon the prunes, mix carefully and bake moderately until done. Place on ice and serve with cream. Add chopped nuts if desired.—Mrs. Fred Smith.

FRUIT COCKTAIL.

Fresh pineapple cut into very small bits, add to this small pieces of orange, banana, grape fruit, lemon juice. Serve in punch glasses with finely chopped ice in it. Two or three whole strawberries on top and powdered sugar, just a little, sprinkled over.—Mrs. Fred Smith.

ORANGE CHARLOTTE.

Line a mold with ladyfingers. Soak one-third box of gelatine in one-third cup of cold water until soft. Pour on one-third cup boiling water, one cup sugar, juice of one lemon. Strain and add one cup orange juice and pulp with a little of the grated rind. Cool in a pan of ice water. Beat the whites of three eggs until very stiff. When the jelly begins to harden beat until very light, then add the whites, beating until stiff. Put in molds and set on ice until time to serve.—Mrs. S. L. Thomas.

SCHAUM TORTE.

Whites of six eggs beaten stiff, add one and one-half cups of granulated sugar and one tablespoonful of vinegar, add a little flavoring if desired. Fold in the sugar. Put in an angel's food pan and bake about one hour in a slow oven, just the same as you bake an angel cake. Serve with whipped cream, with or without fresh fruit.—Mrs. Fred Smith.

ANGEL PARFAIT.

This dessert is novel, yet inexpensive and extremely simple to make. It makes a handsome company dish by the addition of whipped cream above the parfait, sprinkled with chopped pistachio nuts or with candied violets, crushed fine, Boil one cup of sugar and three-fourths of a cup of water until it spins a thread three inches in length. Then pour the sirup in a fine stream on the whites of three eggs, beaten dry. Beat until the mixture is cold. Add a scant tablespoon of vanilla extract and fold in one pint of cream, beaten firm. Turn the mixture into a mold or the can of a freezer, cover securely to avoid salt water, surround with equal measures of salt and crushed ice. Let stand two hours or longer, renewing the salt and ice if needed. When lightly and evenly frozen fill the glasses.—Mrs. Sears.

LEMON ICE.

One quart new milk, one pint granulated sugar, juice of three lemons. Stir the lemon juice into the milk, then stir in sugar and freeze. The milk will thicken at once when lemon juice is added, similar to the effect produced by a junket tablet.—Mrs. Edyth E. Stacks.

RAISIN PUFFS.

Two eggs, one-half cup butter, one cup sweet milk, three teaspoonfuls baking powder, two cups flour, one cup seeded raisins. Steam three-quarters of an hour in buttered cups. When done turn from the cups and serve hot with sauce.

Sauce.—Mix tablespoonful cornstarch with one cup sugar, stir into one pint of boiling water. Let boil ten minutes, then add butter size of a large walnut, tablespoonful vinegar or currant jelly and vanilla.—Mrs. F. E. Frazier.

PEACH FROST.

Take one dozen ripe peaches, peel and slice fine, one cup sugar, one pint rich sweet cream. Mix well and freeze.—Miss Geiken.

DATE WHIP.

Soak one cup tapioca one-half hour in luke-warm water. whites of five eggs, one-fourth teaspoonful cream tartar, one-half cup sugar. Stone the dates, chop fine and cook to a paste in the hot water. Beat the whites of eggs until foamy, add one-fourth spoonful cream of tartar and beat until dry, then add sugar to date paste gradually. Bake in buttered pan set in dish of hot water about twenty-five minutes. Serve with whipped cream or custard sauce—Mrs. F. E. Cartier.

TAPIOCA CREAM.

Soak one cup tapioca one-half hour in luke-warm water. Put one pint sweet milk into a double boiler, let it get scalding hot, then add one cup sugar and the soaked tapioca. Let cook until tapioca becomes clear. Beat the yolks of two eggs with a little milk and add to the pudding. Beat the whites to a stiff froth, add one-half of them to the pudding, beating it up well. Flavor with vanilla. Sweeten the remaining whites and put on top.—Mrs. L. W. Van Dusen.

CRANBERRY FRAPPE.

Boil one quart of cranberries in one pint of water for five or six minutes, strain through a coarse cheesecloth, add one pint of sugar and stir; boil until the sugar is dissolved; when cold add the strained juice of two lemons. Freeze to a mush, using equal parts of ice and salt. Serve in glass cups, either with or just after roast turkey.—Miss Juanita Felts.

MARSHMALLOW SNOW.

One-half cup butter, two and one-fourth cups flour, one water, let boil two minutes and add one tablespoonful of gelatine soaked in one-fourth cupful cold water. Remove from the fire and stir in one-third teaspoonful vanilla and one-fourth teaspoonful pistachio extract. Strain the mixture over the stiffly beaten whites of four eggs, beating all the time. Chill quickly and heap roughly in a serving dish. Upon the beating depends the fine grains of snow.

FRENCH CREAM.

Three tablespoonfuls of grated apple, drain off the juice. The white of one egg, one cup of sugar. Put in a large bowl and beat one-half hour. When very light add one teaspoonful of vanilla, set on ice. Serve with whipped cream.—Lilian Compton.

SNOW BALLS.

One-half cup butter, two and one-fourth cups flour, one cup sugar, three teaspoonfuls baking powder, one-half cup milk, whites of four eggs. Cream butter and sugar. Gradually add milk, then flour sifted with baking powder, and last the whites of eggs beaten stiff. Steam thirty-five minutes in buttered cups. Serve with preserved fruit or strawberry sauce.—Mrs. Susan F. Thomas.

CHARLOTTTE RUSSE.

One pint of cream whipped stiff, one-fourth ounce gelatine dissolved in one-half gill hot milk, whites of two eggs beaten to a froth, one cup powdered sugar, flavor to taste with vanilla. Whip the cream very light, add eggs with which sugar and flavoring have been mixed. Stir in gelatine last as it must be cool. Line bottom of a glass dish with macaroons, pour mixture over them, then dot the top with macaroons.—Mrs. Fred Smith.

SPANISH CREAM.

One-quarter box of gelatine soaked in a little cold water, heat one pint of milk, put in gelatine, stirring until dissolved. Take yolks of three eggs, one-half cup of sugar, one-half teaspoonful of salt beaten well and added to milk; let boil for a few minutes, but not curdle. Remove from fire and add the whites of eggs well beaten. Pour into a mold wet with water, then put in a cool place.—Mrs. F. M. Harris.

STRAWBERRY FLOAT.

Beat one cup of sugar, the white of one egg and one cup crushed strawberries together for fifteen minutes. One hour before serving add one-half cup of cream whipped stiff and one quart of whole berries and place on ice to get cold. —Miss Geiken.

FAIRY DESSERT.

Put a tumbler of jelly into saucepan, add one cup boiling water, stir until melted and at boiling point. Add two tablespoonfuls cornstarch mixed with one-quarter saltspoonful of salt and one-quarter cup cold water. Cook until clear and smooth, then let cook slowly for ten minutes. Turn into large bowl and when cold and beginning to stiffen beat long and hard with egg beater till quite light. Then add beaten whites of two eggs and beat until feathery mass. Turn into wet molds. When stiff and cold serve with whipped cream.—Mrs. H. A. Putnam.

DAINTY DESSERT.

One package each of strawberry and lemon jello. Dissolve according to directions. Put half the strawberry in a common bar cake tin. When stiff sprinkle over slightly broken walnut meats, then the cold lemon and more walnuts, and when stiff the remainder of the strawberry. Slice as you would cake and serve with whipped cream.—Mrs. Cruickshank.

MARSHMALLOW DESSERT.

One pound marshmallows cut in four pieces, one pound raisins cut in two, ten cents worth of pecans and walnuts; cream, flavored with vanilla, enough to cover this. Let stand twenty-four hours. Serve with whipped cream and a cherry.—Winnifred M. Rice.

CHOCOLATE ARROW-ROOT BLANC MANGE (My Own).

One pint sweet milk, about one-eighth of a cake of Baker's chocolate, one and a half tablespoonfuls of powdered arrow-root, dissolved in a little milk; let the milk come to a boil, add the chocolate and arrow-root and stir until thick, then turn into mould, and when cold serve with cream and sugar. This is especially good for invalids.—Mrs. E. H. Green.

SAILOR DUFF.

One egg, two tablespoonfuls sugar, two tablespoonfuls butter, one-half cup molasses, one and one-half cups flour, one teaspoonful soda, one-half cup boiling water. Steam one hour.—Mrs. Fred Smith.

SAINT CECILIA SAUCE.

Yolks of two eggs, one cup of sugar, one cup of cream; beat the yolks and sugar together then add the beaten cream. Flavor with vanilla.—Mrs. Fred Smith.

CHARLOTTE RUSSE.

Four eggs, one ounce of gelatine, one-half pound of sugar, one pint of milk, one quart of cream. Beat yolks with sugar, the whites separately, dissolve the gelatine in the pint of milk, season with vanilla. Add the ingredients. Beat them well. Whip the cream to a froth and add to the mixture. Line two moulds with sponge cake and pour the mixture over it. Set in a cool place until it stiffens.—Helen M. Meech.

LEMON ICE.

One quart fresh milk, one pint sugar. When half frozen add the juice of three lemons.—Mrs. Archibald Buttars.

STRAWBERRY SHORTCAKE.

One pint of flour, two teaspoonfuls Royal Baking Powder, one-half cup butter, one pint sweet milk. Rub butter in flour, then stir with spoon. Add milk so that the butter will spread smoothly. Bake in two pans, butter; add berries, or one can of pineapple, six oranges cut fine, two cups of sugar. Serve with cream.—Mrs. LeFevre.

CUP BLANC MANGE.

Put one pint rich milk in double boiler, add a pinch of salt, stir three tablespoonfuls of sugar and two dessertspoonfuls of cornstarch into one-half cup of milk, add to the milk when scalding hot. Cook five minutes, then add the stiffly beaten whites of two eggs. Remove from the fire and turn into five small cups previously dipped in cold water.—Margaret L. Washburn.

NUT CONSERVE.

Take three pints of any good fruit juice (grape preferred). To each pint of juice add a pound of sugar, six oranges, sliced thin (seeds removed), juice and grated rind of two lemons, two pounds of raisins, stoned and chopped, one pound of English walnuts, kernels coarsely chopped, and one-half pound chopped filberts. Put fruit juice and sugar on to heat. When sugar is dissolved add slowly the other ingredients and cook for one hour, or until it becomes about like marmalade. Seal in small jars. It will be found a rich and delicious sweetmeat. An old, tried English recipe.

Tart apples or berry dumplings are much improved by putting them in a deep dish so that they can be nearly covered with boiling water and generously sprinkled with sugar. Bake until the water and sugar form a syrup.—Mrs. Geo. F. Brown, Daytona, Fla.

CHOCOLATE CUSTARD.

One pint of milk, three ounces of chocolate. Boil this with five tablespoonfuls of sugar till thoroughly mixed, then take off the fire and while hot, add four eggs beaten light. When cold add one pint cream beaten stiff.—Mrs. O. A. Sears.

MAPLE PARFAIT.

One cup maple syrup, four eggs, one tablespoonful gelatine, one pint whipped cream. Cook egg yolks and syrup in double boiler. Cool, then add cream and beaten whites. Pack in mold and freeze in salted ice.—Mrs. O. A. Sears.

ICE CREAM—(Very Fine).

One pint cream, one cup milk, one cup sugar, one egg beaten light, two teaspoonfuls vanilla.—May Guyles Bailey

FRENCH CREAM.

Three tablespoonfuls grated apple, drain off the juice white of one egg, one cup sugar. Put in a large bowl and beat one-half hour. When very light add one teaspoonful vanilla. Set on ice. Serve with whipped cream.—Lillian Compton.

PRUNE WHIP.

Twenty prunes boiled and mashed, whites of six eggs beaten stiff, add one scant cup of sugar, then prunes. Serve with whipped cream.—Miss Mabel Buttars.

MILK SHERBET.

Two quarts fresh milk, juice of four large lemons, four cups sugar. Put into freezer and after freezing a short time add a meringue made of the whites of two eggs and two tablespoonfuls of sugar.—Mrs. John S. Rood.

CREAM DESSERT.

Ten cents worth of dates, ten cents worth of figs, ten cents wortth of walnut meats, ten cents worth of marshmallows. Cut these with scissors and stir them into one pint of cream whipped stiff and sweetened a little.—Mrs. A. F. Bridge.

PINEAPPLE PARFAIT.

One cup pineapple juice, one cup sugar, two tablespoonfuls lemon juice, one tablespoonful gelatine, dissolved in one-fourth cup water. Let this cool until it thickens, then add one and one-half or one pint whipped cream. Mold and freeze.—Mrs.O. A. Sears.

GRAPE FRUIT SHERBET.

Take out the pulp of two large grape fruit, cut them in pieces and crush them to extract the juice. Into a bowl put one pound of granulated sugar and add, a little at a time, one pint of cold water stirring constantly. Add this to the fruit pulp, cover the bowl and allow it to stand two hours, then strain. If it becomes hard to force the pulp through the sieve, add a small cupful of cold water to ease it. Put the mixture, after straining, together with the juice of three large oranges into the freezer and freeze. Leave in freezer one hour. This should not be as stiff as ice cream.—Florence M. Smith.

APPLE FRITTERS.

Make a batter of one cup sweet milk, two cups flour, one heaping teaspoonful baking powder, two eggs, beaten separately, one tablespoonful sugar, a little salt. Have the milk slightly heated, add slowly to the beaten yolks and sugar, then the flour and whites of eggs. Add slices of sour apple. Drop in boiling lard by the spoonful with apple in each one, and fry to a light brown. Serve with maple syrup. —Lillian Compton.

PEACH WHIP.

Press one large mellow peach through a sieve into a deep bowl, add white of one egg and one-fourth pint of sugar, beat until very light. Chill and serve on squares of sponge cake.—Mrs. Noble.

ICE-CREAM SANDWICHES.

Cut ice cream into thin slices with a sharp knife and lay it between firm pieces of sponge cake. Pack on ice until the moment of serving. Very dainty and delicate. Any of the sweet wafers make a good ice cream sandwich.—Mrs. Robert Davidson.

Mr Ogdens long keeping
Catsup
Scald and peel Tomatoes
And lay in Preserving Kettle
without water.
add 3-Raw Onions.
Cook untill done and put
through sieve.
to each gallon of strained
Tomatto. add.
1 cup sugar.
2½ " Vinegar
1 table spoon of salt
1 tea " Black pepper
½ " " Red "
1 " " cloves.
1 " " allspice
1 cinnamon
boil all togather one hour and
bottle hot. Oct 3-1913

July 29-1919

Conserve

Mrs Hemingways Gooseberry Conserve

6 qts green Gooseberrys
2 lbs seeded Raisins
5 " Gran sugar.
4 or 5 Oranges. Juice of all and rind of 3.

Cook the peal in boiling water. Changeing the water once or twice and cook untill tender. Cook Ingredients togather untill right consistency

Cream Puffs

Melt ½ cup Butter in 1 Cup
of boiling water. stir in
1 Cup of Sifted flour.
take from the fire and
when Cool. stir in 3 Eggs
one at a time
bake in little gem tins
in quite a hot oven. 30 m
when cold cut hole in the side
of the top and fill with
whipped cream or custard
E. S.

Mock Angel Cake

Put one cup of milk on
stove in basin. let come
to a boil. take 1½ cups flour
one cup sugar.
3 teaspoons B. Powder. sift
4 times than pour hot
milk in and mix smooth
than fold in whites of
3 eggs beaten stiff
Do not grease tin.
E. S.

IN all receipts in this book calling for baking powder use "Royal." Better and finer food will be the result, and you will safeguard it against alum.

In receipts calling for one teaspoonful of soda and two of cream of tartar, use two spoonfuls of Royal, and leave the cream of tartar and soda out. You get the better food and save much trouble and guess work.

Look out for alum baking powders. Do not permit them to come into your house under any consideration. They add an injurious substance to your food, destroying in part its digestibility. All doctors will tell you this, and it is unquestionable. The use of alum in whiskey is absolutely prohibited; why not equally protect the food of our women and children?

Alum baking powders may be known by their price. Baking powders at a cent an ounce or ten or twenty-five cents a pound are made from alum. Avoid them. Use no baking powder unless the label shows it is made from cream of tartar.

CAKES.

Pat-a-cake, pat-a-cake, to please the men,
Who always like cake until after—when?
Slip in the oven and bake golden brown,
Ice it, and slice it, and capture the town.

CHOCOLATE CAKE.

One cup of butter and two cups of sugar creamed together. Three cups of flour sifted twice with two teaspoonfuls of baking powder. Two-thirds cup of sweet milk or cold water put in alternately with the flour. Whites of six eggs beaten thoroughly; put in just before baking. Flavor with vanilla and bake in five layers.

Filling.—Two full cups of sugar and three-fourths cup of boiling water. Cook together very quickly until it ropes like candy; stir while cooking. Pour this hot syrup very slowly into four well-beaten yolks of eggs. Add immediately two-thirds cup of grated Baker's chocolate. Flavor with vanilla and stir vigorously until creamy and cool enough to put on the cake.—Mrs. James S. Wright.

CHOCOLATE CAKE.

One-half cup butter, one-half cup of sugar, two eggs, one-half cup milk. Mix four ounces chocolate in one-half cup of boiling water, two cups of flour with one teaspoonful baking powder.—Mrs. F. M. Harris.

DEVIL'S FOOD CAKE.

Cream one-fourth cup butter, add one cup sugar, and cream until very light, beat in two whole eggs, one teaspoon soda in half cup thick sour milk, one-half teaspoon baking powder in one and a quarter cups of flour, break one-fourth cake Baker's chocolate in cup and add enough boiling water to make cup half full, and add to cake the last thing. Flavor with vanilla.

Icing for Above.—One-half cup granulated sugar, one-half cup water, boil until it hairs; add three marshmallows and stir smooth, then stir into it the beaten white of one egg. Beat until thick enough to spread. Let it set on cake, then pour over the white icing the following: One-fourth cake Baker's chocolate melted, add piece of butter size of walnut.—Mrs. John S. Rood.

CHOCOLATE CAKE.

Two cups of sugar, one-half cup of butter, one cup of sweet milk, whites of six eggs beaten very light, three cups of flour and two teaspoonfuls of baking powder.

Frosting.—Whites of two eggs beaten to a stiff froth. one cup of powdered sugar, about one-eighth of a cake of Baker's chocolate; boil in water from ten to fifteen minutes and spread over the cake.—May Guyles Bailey.

MARBLE CHOCOLATE CAKE.

One cup of butter, two small cups of sugar, four well-beaten eggs, one cup of sweet milk, three cups of flour, two teaspoonfuls baking powder. Take one cup of this batter and mix with four tablespoonfuls of grated chocolate, dissolved in a little cream, drop as for marble cake.—Mrs. Mary Yettaw.

DEVIL CAKE.

Two cups brown sugar, one-half cup butter mix together; three eggs, one-half cup boiling water and dissolve one-fourth cake chocolate, one-half cup sour milk, one large teaspoon soda, three cups flour, one-half teaspoon baking powder.

Frosting.—One and one-half cups brown sugar, scant one-half cup butter, one-half cup sweet milk. Boil ten minutes, then add one teaspoon vanilla. Cool and stir.—Mrs. Grace Hyers.

DEVIL'S FOOD.

Grate one cup Baker's chocolate or three tablespoons of cocoa, yolk of one egg, one-half cup of sweet milk one-half cup of sugar. Cook until thick, then cool.

Two-thirds cup of sugar, one egg, one tablespoon melted butter, one-half cup sweet milk, one and one-half cups of flour, one teaspoon of soda, one teaspoon of baking powder. Put soda and baking powder in flour, then mix two parts together and bake in three layers.—Mrs. Frank Hull.

ANGEL CAKE.

Boil until it threads: One and one-half cups sugar with four tablespoons of water. Pour over the beaten whites of eleven eggs. When rather cool, fold in gently, one cup well-sifted flour, one teaspoon cream tartar, one teaspoon corn starch. Flavor and salt. Bake in slow oven forty minutes. —Emily E. Jefferies.

DEVIL'S FOOD CAKE.

Melt over fire one cup grated chocolate, one cup brown sugar, one-half cup sweet milk; cool and add yolk of one egg, well beaten, then set aside. Cream one cup brown sugar with one-half cup butter, add one-half cup milk and yolks of two eggs, then two cups of flour and fold in stiffly beaten whites of two eggs. Lastly add one teaspoon soda dissolved in a little warm water. Melt over tea kettle five cents' worth of marshmallows, boil until it threads; one cup sugar and one-half cup of water with one teaspoon white vinegar; beat remaining white of egg stiff and add syrup and marshmallows; stir until it becomes thick and put between layers.—Mrs. Marting.

DEVILS CAKE.

Four tablespoons of cocoa, yolk of one egg, one-half cup of milk, one-half cup of sugar. Cook until thick, then cool.

Beat separately two-thirds cup of sugar, one egg, one tablespoon of melted butter, one-half cup of milk, one and one-half cups of flour, one teaspoon soda, one teaspoon of baking powder. Put the soda and baking powder in flour and sift; then mix the two batters together, and bake in three layers.—Cora Cook.

DEVILS FOOD.

One-half cake of chocolate melted in steam, one cup of milk stirred in chocolate; set this to one side. Two cups of pulverized sugar, one-half cup of butter; mix well, then add yolks of four eggs, leaving out two whites for icing. Stir in the milk and chocolate one teaspoonful of vanilla, two heaping cups of flour, two teaspoonfuls of baking powder. Beat the whites of two eggs and stir in lastly.—Miss Jaunita Felts.

DEVILS FOOD CAKE.

One cup sugar, one tablespoon butter, yolks of three eggs, well beaten; one and one-half squares chocolate, melted; one-half cup sweet milk, two teaspoons baking powder, one and one-half cups flour, and lastly whites of two eggs well beaten. Bake quickly.—Mrs. H. R. Fowler.

SPONGE CAKE.

Four egg whites and yolks beaten separately, three-fourths cup sugar, four tablespoons cold water, one cup flour before sifting, one-half teaspoon baking powder.—Mrs. O. A. Sears.

ANGEL FOOD.

Whites of nine large or ten small eggs, one and one-fourth cups sugar (measure after sifting), one cup flour (measure after sifting), one-half teaspoon cream of tartar, pinch of salt added to eggs before beating. Add cream of tartar when eggs are half beaten. Sift sugar and flour three or four times, then measure. Sift sugar, then flour, into beaten eggs. Add one-half teaspoonful vanilla and one-half teaspoonful lemon extract. Put in an ungreased tin and bake forty minutes in slow oven.—Mrs. A. L. Coulter.

CHOCOLATE SPONGE.

Three tablespoons butter, seven-eighths cup sugar, yolks three eggs beaten stiff, one teaspoon cinnamon, four tablespoons cocoa, one-half cup water, one and three-eighths cups flour, two teaspoons baking powder, one-half teaspoon vanilla, whites of three eggs stiffly beaten.

Chocolate Frosting.—One cup sugar, one-third cup boiling water, one and one-half squares chocolate, one-half teaspoon vanilla.—A Friend.

CREAM SPONGE CAKE.

Put two eggs in cup, then fill cup with cream and beat. Add one cup sugar (beat), one and one-half cups flour, one teaspoonful soda and cream tartar. Pinch of salt and vanilla.—Mrs. F. M. Harris.

SPONGE CAKE.

Three eggs, one and one-half cups flour, one and one-half cups sugar, one-half cup cold water, a little salt, rind and juice of one-half lemon, two small teaspoons baking powder or (one-half soda and one cream tartar). Beat yolks with a little of the water and sugar quickly, then part of flour. Put cream of tartar in last of the flour and soda in last of water. Add whites last. Bake in a slow oven.—Mrs. (Dr.) Armstrong.

DOLLY VARDEN CAKE.

Two cups sugar, two-thirds butter creamed, three eggs beaten thoroughly, one cup milk, three cups flour, three teaspoons baking powder, one cup chopped raisins, one-half cup currants, one piece finely chopped citron. Take half the dough, add one spoon molasses and the fruit. Bake in layers and place alternately together. Fill with any nice filling and frost.—Mrs. Edyth E. Stacks.

HOT WATER SPONGE CAKE.

One cup of sugar and two eggs beaten until very light. Add one teaspoonful of baking powder sifted with one cup of flour. Stir well together, then add one-third cup of boiling water and bake in a deep cake tin, that has been buttered and floured, in a moderate oven.—Mrs. Rose Taylor.

VELVET SPONGE CAKE.

Beat two eggs very light, then stir in one cup of granulated or powdered sugar; next stir in one cup of sifted flour with two teaspoonfuls of baking powder; then add gradually one-half cup of boiling water. Flavor and bake in a well heated oven.—Mrs. F. Wood.

FRUIT CAKE.

Two cups of brown sugar, one cup butter, one cup molasses, one cup strong coffee, four eggs, one teaspoon soda, two teaspoons cinnamon, cloves, one teaspoon nutmeg, one pound raisins, one pound currants, one pound English walnuts, four and one-half cups flour, one-half pound of candied fruits, lemon, orange, citron, pineapple and candied cherries.—Mrs. Will Johnson.

WHITE FRUIT CAKE.

One cup sugar, one-half cup butter, one egg, one cup milk, two cups sifted flour, two teaspoons baking powder, one-half cup cocoanut, one-half cup almonds, one-half cup citron, a little orange and lemon peel. Bake in sheets and cut in squares.—Lillian Compton.

SULTANA CAKE.

One-half pound butter, one-half pound sugar, four eggs, three-fourths pound flour, one-half teaspoonful baking powder, one half pound Sultana raisins, one-fourth pound orange peel, a few drops of lemon extract. Beat the butter and sugar together. Add eggs, then flour with baking powder, then raisins and peel. Bake in a moderate oven one hour. —Mrs. John A. Crawford.

DRIED APPLE CAKE.

Two cups dried apples chopped fine and soaked over night. Then cook in one cup of molasses until tender. Add one cup sugar, one cup butter, one cup sour milk, one teaspoonful each of cinnamon, cloves and lemon extract, one nutmeg, two teaspoons soda, flour to make a stiff batter. Bake in moderate oven. One cup of raisins may be added. —Mrs. A. Ross.

SPONGE CAKE.

One cup of sugar, three eggs well beaten, three tablespoons sweet milk, one teaspoon lemon extract, one cup of flour, two teaspoons baking powder.—Mrs. W. E. Bedwin.

SPONGE CAKE.

Six eggs, three-fourths pint granulated sugar, one pint flour. Beat the eggs, adding sugar slowly, then add flour. Stir just enough to mix. Flavor with lemon.—Miss Honor Nicholls.

POTATO CAKE.

One cup of butter, two cups of sugar, one cup of mashed potato, one-half cup of sweet milk or coffee, one cup of chopped nuts or raisins, three cups of flour, four eggs, one teaspoon of cinnamon, one nutmeg, two teaspoons of baking powder.—Mrs. F. L. Higbee.

EAGLE CAKE.

One cup of brown sugar, one-half cup of butter, one cup of sour milk, one cup of chopped raisins, two cups of flour, one egg, one tablespoon of molasses, one teaspoon of soda, one-half teaspoon of cinnamon, one-fourth teaspoon of cloves, one-half nutmeg. Bake in a slow oven.

—Miss Hutchinson.

BUTTERMILK CAKE.

Two cups of sugar, one-half cup of butter, one egg, two cups of buttermilk, two cups of chopped raisins, one teaspoon each of cloves, cinnamon, allspice and nutmeg, four cups of flour, two teaspoons soda.—Mrs. W. E. Bedwin.

DAINTY FRUIT CAKE.

Two cups dates and two cups of walnuts chopped, one cup sugar, four eggs, whites and yolks beaten separately, one teaspoonful baking powder in six tablespoonfuls flour. —Mrs. John S. Rood.

PORK CAKE.

Take one pound of fat salt pork, free from lean or rind. Chop as fine as to be almost like lard. Pour upon it one-half pint of boiling water. Add two cups of sugar, a teaspoonful of soda stirred into one cup of molasses, one pound of raisins, one-fourth pound of citron shaved fine, and enough flour to make of the consistency of common cake batter. Season with one teaspoonful each of cloves and nutmeg and two of cinnamon. Bake in a moderate oven.—Mrs. Rose Taylor.

WHITE FRUIT CAKE.

Three-fourths cup butter, two cups sugar, one cup sweet milk, two and one-half cups flour, two teaspoons baking powder, four eggs beaten separately, half cup more of flour mixed with baking powder, one cup seedless raisins, one cup of English walnuts, one-fourth pound citron. Flavor with almond. Bake slowly one hour.—Mrs. Todd.

HICKORY NUT CAKE.

One and one-half cups sugar, one-half cup butter, two eggs, three-fourths cup sweet milk, two cups flour, one cup nuts chopped fine, warmed and sprinkled with a little flour, one teaspoon soda and two cream tartar.—Mrs. R. J. Walters.

FRUIT CAKE WITHOUT EGGS.

One teaspoonful soda in two tablespoonfuls warm water; add to this one cup thick sour cream or one-half cup sour milk and one-half cup shortening, one-half cup molasses, one cup brown sugar, one tablespoonful cinnamon, one pound raisins-currants, one cup chopped citron, and flour to make very stiff. (This makes two large loaf cakes.)—

FRUIT CAKE WITHOUT MOLASSES.

Two cups brown sugar, two-thirds cup butter, spice to suit taste. Four eggs beaten, one cup sour cream in which one teaspoon soda is dissolved. One pound each of raisins and currants, one-half cup each of citron and lemon peel chopped very fine. One cup walnut meats chopped fine, three cups flour. Add flour and fruit alternately.—Lillian Compton.

PLAIN FRUIT CAKE.

Two cups brown sugar, one and one-half cups butter, one cup molasses, six eggs, one cup sweet milk, one teaspoon soda, one and one-half pounds raisins, one pound currants, one-fourth pound orange peel, one teaspoonful nutmeg and cinnamon, four cups flour, using one to sift over fruit named to prevent fruit falling. Vanilla. Cook in moderate oven.—Mrs. F. M. Harris.

WHITE FRUIT CAKE.

One cup of sugar, one-half cup of butter, beat to a cream; one-half cup of sweet milk, whites of four eggs beaten very light, two and one-half cups of flour, one-half teaspoon of soda and one of cream tartar, or two teaspoons of baking powder, one pound of raisins chopped. Measure in a coffee cup.—Mrs. John Nicholls.

ECONOMY CAKE.

One cup butter, two cups sugar, one cup chopped raisins, one cup sour milk, three cups flour, one teaspoon soda, two eggs, all kinds of spices to taste.—Mrs. John O. Miller.

FRUIT CAKE.

Two cups of brown sugar, one-half cup of butter, one cup of sour milk, two and one-half scant cups of flour, yolks of two eggs, one teaspoonful soda, one cup of raisins, one cup of nut meats, spices.—Mrs. L. E. Benton.

SPICE CAKE.

One tablespoon butter, one cup buttermilk, one cup brown sugar, one teaspoon nutmeg, one teaspoon cinnamon, one teaspoon allspice, one cup chopped raisins, one egg, one teaspoon soda. Not too stiff.—Mrs. Arthur L. Fitch.

DRIED APPLE OR FARMER'S FRUIT CAKE.

Soak in water three cups of dried apples over night; chop lightly in the morning and let them simmer two hours in two cups of molasses (black strap), add two eggs, one cup sugar, one cup sweet milk, three-fourths cup butter, two teaspoons soda, and flour to make a stiff batter. Spice to suit the taste. Bake in a moderate oven. This makes a large cake, or three common sized loaf cakes.—Mrs. F. E. Frazier.

FRUIT CAKE.

One and one-half pounds butter, one and three-fourths pounds sugar, one and three-fourths pounds flour, fifteen eggs, four pounds raisins, four pounds currants, two pounds citron, two nutmegs, cloves, cinnamon and allspice. Bake two and one-half or three hours.—Mrs. A. L. Coulter.

NUT SLICES.

One pound brown sugar, five eggs beaten light with sugar, two squares chocolate (grated), one-fourth pound blanched almonds (chopped), five cents worth citron (chopped), rind of one lemon, one teaspoon cinnamon, half teaspoon cloves, one-fourth teaspoon allspice, flour enough to make a batter that will run in pan. Bake in large dripping pan so it will be quite thin when baked. Cut in squares.—Mrs. R. W. Paddock.

"NEVER FAIL" LAYER CAKE.

Two cups sugar, one-half cup butter, one cup sweet milk, three cups flour, three teaspoons baking powder, whites of four eggs, beaten stiff.—Mrs. H. L. Iddings.

DARK LAYER CAKE.

One-half cup sugar, one-half cup syrup (dark or light), two-thirds cup water, one and two-thirds cups flour, one egg, butter size of egg, one-half teaspoon cloves, one-half teaspoon cinnamon, one teaspoon soda.

Filling.—One cup sugar, one-fourth cup water, white of one egg, raisins. Boil until it "threads" pour on beaten white of one egg, beat while pouring; add chopped raisins, figs or dates.—Mrs. M. N. LaPier.

LAYER CAKE.

One cup of sugar, six tablespoonfuls melted butter, seven tablespoonfuls sweet milk, one and one-half cups of flour, two heaping teaspoons baking powder; lastly, three eggs well beaten.—Mrs. J. Timmer.

FRUIT LAYER CAKE.

One cup of brown sugar, one-half cup of butter, one-half cup of sour milk, two cups of flour, one cup of chopped raisins, large tablespoon of molasses, yolks of two eggs, spice.—Mrs. W. W. Srigley.

SPICE CAKE.

One-half cup each of butter and lard, two cups brown sugar, one-half cup buttermilk, four eggs, one tablespoon spice, one teaspoon soda, two and one-half cups flour.—Mrs. John C. Miller.

SPICE CAKE.

One-half cup butter, one cup sugar, two eggs well beaten, one-half cup sour milk and cream, one-half teaspoon soda, two cups flour, one teaspoon cinnamon, one-half teaspoon cloves, one-half cup raisins, a little nutmeg.—Mrs. R. B. Armstrong.

SPICE CAKE.

One egg, four tablespoons melted butter, two tablespoons molasses in cup and fill with sour milk, one teaspoon soda, one cup sugar, two cups flour, three teaspoons cinnamon, two teaspoons cloves, one teaspoon baking powder.—Mrs. Frank Payne.

SPICE CAKE.

One cup sugar, one cup butter, one cup sour milk, one-half cup molasses, two cups fruit, one cup nut meats, three eggs, one teaspoon each of cinnamon, cloves, soda, and baking powder, add nutmeg and salt. Stir in enough flour to make rather stiff batter. Bake slowly.—Emily E. Jefferies.

SPICE CAKE.

Three eggs, one cup sugar, spices to suit taste, one-half cup lard and butter creamed together, one-half cup black molasses, one cup sour milk, and one teaspoon (big) of soda dissolved in a tablespoon of hot water. Flour enough to make quite a thin batter. Save two egg whites for frosting, and bake in layers.—Mrs. Bert Van Allsburg.

MOLASSES CAKE.

One cup of molasses, two cups of flour, one-half cup of sugar, yolk of one egg, two rounded tablespoons butter melted, one teaspoonful each of cinnamon, cloves, nutmeg, soda and vinegar; pinch of salt. Mix thoroughly and pour over one cup of boiling water. Bake in two layers and make the boiled frosting of the white of the egg and one cup of sugar.—Mrs. Blodgett.

MOLASSES CAKE.

Three-fourths cup New Orleans molasses, three-fourths cup sugar, one egg, two tablespoonfuls melted butter, one teaspoonful each of cinnamon and nutmeg, one-half teaspoonful cloves, pinch of salt, one teaspoonful vinegar, one teaspoonful lemon extract, one cup chopped raisins, all the flour that can be stirred in. Put one teaspoonful soda in a cup of boiling water and pour over. Stir until smooth and bake in a moderate oven. Boiled icing.—Mrs. S. F. Alcox.

PORK CAKE.

One cup fresh pork chopped fine, two cups buttermilk, one and one-half cups brown sugar, one-half cup New Orleans molasses, two cups raisins, two cups currants, and a little grated orange peel; one teaspoon soda, a pinch of salt. Mix pork well in buttermilk first and flour enough to make ordinary cake batter. If kept in a stone crock, will become better with age.—Mrs. Hattie J. Cooper.

PORK CAKE.

One pound chopped pork, two cups of sugar, one and one-half cups of cold coffee, two eggs, two cups raisins, two teaspoons soda, spice to taste, and flour for sufficient batter. —Mrs. Lynn.

SUNSHINE CAKE.

Three eggs, one cup sugar, one cup flour, one teaspoonful lemon, one teaspoonful baking powder, two tablespoonfuls boiling water.—Mrs. F. M. Harris.

PORK CAKE.

One pound currants, one pound raisins, one ounce lemon peel, one teaspoon cloves and cinnamon, one nutmeg, one cup molasses, one cup brown sugar, one pound pork chopped fine, one pint boiling water poured on the pork, one teaspoon salt, flour enough to mix stiff.—Mrs. Wm. Scroggie.

WHITE CAKE.

One egg, one cup of sugar, butter size of egg, one cup of sweet milk, two teaspoons of baking powder, flour.—Mrs. W. W. Srigley.

SUNSHINE CAKE.

Six eggs, one cup of granulated sugar, one cup of flour well sifted, one teaspoon of cream tartar; beat yolks of eggs well; beat whites of eggs about half, then sift in cream tartar and beat till stiff. Add sugar and beat a minute. Then blend in yolks; do not beat. Add flour gradually and stir as little as possible. Bake one hour in a slow oven. —Miss Hutchinson.

MRS. PARMELEE'S CAKE.

One and one-half cups sugar, one-half cup butter, one-half cup milk, full measure; three eggs, leaving one-half the white of one for frosting; two teaspoons baking powder, two cups of flour (before sifting). Sift flour and baking powder together.

FEATHER CAKE.

Four eggs, beaten separately; one and one-quarter cups granulated sugar, three-quarters cup butter, one-half cup water, two and one-half cups swansdown cake flour, two teaspoons baking powder, flavor to taste. Sift flour once, then measure; add baking powder and sift three times; cream, butter and sugar thoroughly; beat yolks to a very stiff froth and stir in; whip whites until very stiff; add water, then whites of eggs, then flour, then flavor and stir very hard. Put in slow oven at once; will bake in thirty to forty minutes. Good for layers; any kind of light filling.

QUICK LOAF CAKE.

One pound of flour, three-quarters pound of sugar, one-half pound of butter, three eggs well beaten, one teaspoonful vanilla, one cup of sweet milk, two teaspoons of baking powder sifted into the flour, large cup of raisins (more if desired), one-half nutmeg.—Mrs. John Nicholls.

CUP CAKE.

One egg, one cup sugar, one cup sour milk, one teaspoon baking soda, one-half cup shortening, one and one-half teaspoons cinnamon, one and one-half teaspoons cloves, one cup chopped raisins, two cups flour.—Mrs. M. E. Ackert.

GOLD (LOAF) CAKE.

Yolks of eight eggs, one and one-half cups granulated sugar, two-thirds cup butter, two-thirds cup sweet milk, two and one-half cups flour, one teaspoon cream of tartar, scant one-half teaspoon soda; sift flour once, then measure; add soda and sift three times. Cream butter and sugar thoroughly. beat yolks a little, then add cream of tartar, beat to a stiff froth; add this to creamed butter and sugar; stir well; add milk; then flour; stir hard; flavor. Put in slow oven and bake thirty to fifty minutes.—Mrs. O. A. Sears.

DELICIOUS CAKE.

Two cups white sugar, one cup butter, one cup milk, three eggs, one teaspoonful soda, two teaspoons cream tartar, three cups sifted flour.—Mrs. W. G. Stevenson.

MARBLE CAKE.

Light part—one and one-half cups sugar, one-half cup butter, one-half cup water, two large cups flour, four whites of eggs, one teaspoon baking powder, one lemon, juice and grated rind.

Dark part—one cup sugar, one-quarter cup butter, one-half cup water, one and one-half cups flour, one teaspoon baking powder, four yolks of eggs, vanilla flavoring, two ounces melted chocolate.—Mrs. Frank Hull.

MARBLE CAKE.

Light part—one-half cup butter, one cup sugar, four whites of eggs, one-half cup milk, one teaspoon lemon extract, one teaspoon Royal Baking powder, one and one-quarter cups flour.

Dark part—One-half cup butter, one cup brown sugar, one-half cup milk, four yolks of eggs, one and one-quarter cups flour, one teaspoon Royal Baking Powder, one teaspoon extract of cloves, one teaspoon extract of cinnamon, one teaspoon extract of allspice. Cream butter and sugar, adding eggs well beaten, and baking powder sifted in flour, then extracts and milk, beating until fine. Put into paper lined tin. Drop the batters alternately into it.—Sybil Cook.

MARBLE CAKE.

White part—Whites of four eggs well beaten, one cup sugar, one-half cup butter, one-half cup sweet milk, two teaspoons baking powder, two and one-half cups of flour.

Dark part—Yolks of four eggs, one cup brown sugar, one-half cup molasses, one-half cup butter, one-half cup sour milk, one and one-half cups flour, one teaspoon cloves, cinnamon and nutmeg; one teaspoon soda dissolved in milk and added after part of the flour is in.—Mrs. Will Johnson.

SPICE CAKE.

Two eggs, one cup brown sugar, one cup sour cream, one-half teaspoon soda, one-half teaspoon cloves, nutmeg and cinnamon, one cup raisins, one-half cup English walnuts cut fine, one and one-half cups of flour.—Mrs. William C. Woolner.

PORK CAKE.

One pound fat pork chopped fine, one-half pint boiling water poured on pork, one teaspoon soda in water, two cups brown sugar, one cup molasses, one pound raisins, one-quarter pound citron, one-half pound currants, one cup nutmeats, teaspoon of spices, flour to make a common cake batter.—Mrs. Henry B. Wood.

IMPERIAL CAKE.

One pound of sugar, one pound of flour, three-fourths pound of butter, one pound of almonds, blanched and cut fine, one-half pound of raisins, rind and juice of one lemon, one nutmeg, ten eggs. This is very delicious and will keep for months.—Mrs. F. J. Meech.

HEAVENLY FOOD.

One cup of dates cut in pieces, one cup of walnut meats broken, two eggs beaten together not very much, three-fourths cup of sugar, three heaping tablespoons of flour, one teaspoon of baking powder. Bake in sheets. Cut up in strips about a finger in length. Can be served for dessert with whipped cream.—Mrs. D. F. Meech.

SCOTCH CAKE.

One pound of flour, one pound of sugar, three-fourths pound of butter, the juice and grated rind of one lemon, nine eggs, one pound of raisins, one teaspoon of baking powder.—Mrs. F. J. Meech.

SOFT MOLASSES GINGERBREAD.

Melt a teacup of butter, mix it with a pint of molasses, a tablespoonful of ginger, a pint of flour and a couple of beaten eggs. Dissolve a couple of teaspoonfuls of soda in one-half pint of milk, and stir into the cake. Add flour to make it the consistency of unbaked pound cake. Bake in deep pans about one-half hour.—Miss L. P. Averill.

COLD-WATER SPONGE CAKE.

Six eggs, three cups of flour, three cups of sugar, one cup of cold water, juice and rind of one lemon, two teaspoons of baking powder. Beat the yolks with the sugar. The whites to a froth. Beat into the yolks and sugar one cup of flour and one-half cup of water; then add second cup of flour and one-half cup of water, the last cup of flour with the baking powder.—Mrs. F. J. Meech.

NUT CAKES.

One cup of butter, two cups of sugar, four eggs well beaten, one cup of sour milk or sour cream, if preferred; one teaspoon of soda, four cups of flour, one cup of chopped walnut meats, one-half cup of raisins. Spice to taste with cinnamon, cloves and nutmeg.—Mrs. D. F. Meech.

ALMOND CAKE.

Two cups of sugar one-half cup of butter, one cup of sweet milk, two and one-half cups of flour, whites of eight eggs, one teaspoon of cream tartar, one-half teaspoon of soda. Mix butter and sugar to a cream; mix other ingredients alternately, putting in the soda last. Bake in layers. Spread each layer with soft frosting and add blanched split almonds about an inch apart on each layer.—Mrs. F. J. Meech.

COCOANUT CAKES.

The whites of four eggs beaten stiff, two cups of pulverized sugar, two cups of shredded cocoanut, four soda crackers rolled very fine, two teaspoons of baking powder. —Mrs. D. F. Meech.

COFFEE CAKE.

Two cups of brown sugar, one cup butter, one cup molasses, one cup strong coffee as prepared for table, four eggs, one teaspoon saleratus, two teaspoons cinnamon, two teaspoons cloves, one teaspoon grated nutmeg, one pound raisins, one pound currants, four cups flour.—Mrs. J. C. Miller.

BREAD CAKE.

One cup sponge, one cup sugar, one egg, one-half cup shortening (butter and lard mixed) one cup flour, one small teaspoon soda, one-half nutmeg.—Mrs. Emma Graves.

GERMAN COFFEE CAKES.

One-fourth cup melted butter, one-half cup granulated sugar, one-half cup sweet milk, two teaspoons baking powder, one scant pint of flour. Mix and roll about one-half inch thick. Sprinkle on the dough three tablespoons granulated sugar mixed with one scant teaspoon cinnamon and roll like a jelly roll. Cut off the thickness of cookies and bake, being careful not to have them too near together in the pan, these are very nice to eat with coffee.—Mrs. H. A. Fowler.

COFFEE CAKE.

Two cups brown sugar, one cup of butter; cream butter and sugar; one cup of New Orleans molasses, one cup of strong coffee as prepared for the table, four eggs well baten, one teaspoon of soda, two teaspoons of cinnamon, two teaspoons of cloves, one teaspoon of grated nutmeg, one cup of raisins, one cup of currants, four cups of flour; sift soda in flour. Bake in slow oven. One-half of this recipe makes a good sized cake.—Mrs. Hattie J. Cooper.

GERMAN COFFEE CAKE.

Three pints bread sponge, three-fourths cup shortening, butter and lard; one cup sugar, one-half nutmeg, one teaspoon salt, one egg. Add sufficient flour to make a soft dough; let rise to twice its size and mix down again; let it come up again, then spread in tins about one-inch thick; let rise very light; before putting in the oven, spread melted butter, cinnamon and sugar. Bake about twenty minutes. —Mrs. G. C. Geiken.

BREAD CAKE.

Cup light dough, two cups sugar, one-half cup melted butter, one cup sweet milk, one egg, one teaspoon soda, one teaspoon cinnamon, one cup raisins. Flour enough to thicken, but not too thick.—Mrs. C. E. See.

LOVELY GINGER BREAD.

One cup brown sugar, one cup butter, two cups molasses, two eggs, two cups buttermilk, five cups flour, two teaspoons ginger; one-half soda. Half of this recipe makes a good sized cake. Very slow oven.—Mrs. F. M. Harris.

JAM CAKE.

Three-fourths cup butter, one cup sugar, one cup jam, one and one-half cups flour, three tablespoons sour cream, one tablespoon soda, one tablespoon cinnamon, one tablespoon nutmeg, two eggs. Blackberry jam preferred. Bake in layers and use boiled icing.—Isabel Hines.

RASPBERRY CAKE.

One-half cup white sugar, two tablespoons of butter and two eggs creamed together; one cup raspberry jam. Stir one teaspoon of soda into the berries and pour into the mixture. Add two cups flour. Bake in layers and put boiled icing between the layers. Canned berries may be used in place of the jam.—Mrs. A. T. Burnett.

..SOFT GINGER BREAD.

One cup brown sugar, one cup molasses, two-thirds cup lard or (one-half butter and one-half lard), one teaspoonful ginger, cinnamon and one-fourth teaspoonful of ground cloves, one teaspoonful soda dissolved in one cup boiling water, two and one-half cups sifted flour, two eggs, a pinch of salt. Mix sugar, molasses and lard thoroughly; add spices and boiling water with soda dissolved in it; stir well; then add flour, and the last thing before putting into cake tin, add two well beaten eggs. Bake in a moderate oven.—Mrs. Glasford.

..SOFT GINGER BREAD.

One egg, one-half cup brown sugar, one-half cup molasses, one-half cup sour milk or buttermilk, one-half tablespoon butter, one-half tablespoon lard, one-half teaspoon cinnamon and ginger. Mix soft.—Mrs. Frank Payne.

FRUIT GINGER BREAD.

One cup molasses, two eggs, well beaten; two teaspoons of soda in a cup of boiling water, cup of chopped raisins, one-half cup of lard, two teaspoons of ginger, one of cinnamon, one-half of cloves, a little salt, two and one-half cups of flour. Bake in a moderate oven. —Mrs. Ward.

..SOFT GINGER BREAD.

One-half cup sugar, one cup molasses, one-half cup butter, one teaspoon ginger, cinnamon and cloves, one teaspoon soda in one cup boiling water, two and one-half cups flour and add two well beaten eggs the last thing before baking.—Mrs. O. D. Hammond.

GINGER CAKE.

One-half cup of sugar, two well beaten eggs, one cup of molasses, one-half cup warm water, one teaspoonful soda, one-half cup lard, one teaspoonful ginger, one-half teaspoonful cloves, a little salt, two cups of flour.—Mrs. Mary Yettaw.

GINGER CAKE.

Two eggs, one cup sugar, one cup sour milk, one tablespoon shortening, one-half cup molasses, one teaspoon soda, two and one-half cups flour; spice.—Mrs. W. J. Stevenson.

ROLL JELLY CAKE (Claire's Favorite).

Cream butter the size of a hickory nut, into one cup granulated sugar, with one-half teaspoon salt and a little grated nutmeg. Add three tablespoonfuls sweet milk. Sift one heaping teaspoonful Royal baking powder with one cup flour. Butter three long baking tins, have a good hot oven; then beat three eggs thoroughly into prepared sugar, beat in the flour and put in oven as quickly as possible. When baked loosen the edge with a thin knife and turn upside down on a folded cloth. Stir jelly smooth, spread on, loosen the cake from tin at one end, roll and loosen as you roll. Place roll in napkin. May also be used for layer cake.—Mary E. Heston.

JELLY ROLL.

One cup of sifted flour, three eggs, one cup of sugar, two tablespoons of water, one teaspoon of baking powder. Beat well, put in a large pan; when baked, put on a damp cloth and roll while warm.—Mrs. John Nicholls.

ROLL JELLY CAKE.

One cup sugar, three eggs well beaten, three tablespoons sweet cream, two teaspoons baking powder, one cup flour. Bake in a shallow dripping pan. When done, spread with jelly and roll in a napkin.—Mrs. Grace Hyres.

SOUR CREAM CAKE.

Two eggs, two cups sugar, one teaspoonful salt, one and one-half cups sour cream, one level teaspoonful soda, two teaspoonfuls baking powder, flavoring.—Mrs. W. H. Woodley.

EGGLESS CAKE.

One cup sugar, one cup sweet milk, two tablespoons butter, two cups flour, one teaspoon baking powder, one-half teaspoon salt.—Mrs. Wm. Scroggie.

ONE EGG CAKE.

One egg, two and one-half cups of flour, two and one-half teaspoonfuls baking powder, one cup of milk, one-half cup butter, one and one-half cups sugar —Mrs. F. M. Sears.

ROLL CAKE.

Three eggs, four tablespoons sugar, one tablespoon baking powder, three tablespoons flour.—Mrs. Wm. Scroggie.

WHITE CAKE.

Whites of three eggs beaten to a froth, one cup white sugar, one-third cup butter, one-half cup sweet milk, one cup flour, one teaspoon baking powder.—Mrs. Arthur Fitch.

WHITE CAKE.

Take two scant cups of sugar, whites of four eggs, two-thirds cup of butter, one cup sweet milk, three cups flour, four teaspoons of baking powder. Flavor to taste.—Mrs. Butler.

ICE CREAM CAKE.

To the whites of five eggs lightly beaten add two cups of sugar, one cup of butter, one cup of milk, three cups of flour and three teaspoonfuls of baking powder. Bake in thin layers and use as a cream to spread between, two and a half cups of sugar and one-half cup of water boiled together. Beat the whites of three eggs to a stiff froth and when the syrup will hair, pour it into the whites and stir as fast as possible. Flavor with lemon and spread between the layers and over top.—Mrs. John Miller.

WHITE CAKE.

Two eggs (one white reserved for frosting), one and one-quarter (scant) cups sugar, one-quarter cup sweet milk, three cups flour, one teaspoon cream of tartar, one-half teaspoon (scant) soda. Flavor to taste. Sift flour once, then measure, add soda, sift three times, cream butter and sugar. Beat eggs, add cream of tartar, then beat thoroughly, add milk, then flour. Bake in two layers; put in slow oven, will bake in fifteen minutes.—Mrs. O. A. Sears.

BLACKBERRY CAKE.

Three eggs, one cup sugar, three-fourths cup butter, one and one-half cups flour, one cup of blackberry jam, three tablespoons of sour cream, one teaspoon each of soda, allspice and cinnamon, one nutmeg; stir well, bake in layers, put icing between.—Mrs. J. T. Olbert.

WHITE LOAF CAKE.

One-half cup granulated sugar, three-fourths cup butter, one cup sweet milk, three cups flour, whites of eight eggs, two teaspoonfuls baking powder, one teaspoonful lemon extract, one teaspoonful vanilla. Cream butter and sugar, add milk, beat whites of eggs and add alternately with flour and baking powder sifted together. Add flavoring and beat all together five minutes. Bake in a moderate oven fifty minutes.—Miss Geiken.

WHITE LOAF CAKE.

One-half cup of butter, cream butter with a fork; add one cup of sugar, one-half a cup of sweet milk, one cup of flour; then put two teaspoonfuls baking powder in same cup and fill with flour, add and beat cake until fine; then add the whites of three eggs well beaten, one teaspoonful vanilla.—Mrs. W. E. Bedwin.

Mrs H. L. Barnum
Sept 12-1914

Olive Oil Pickles

Take Cucumbers the size
of a quarter. wash and
slice. as for the table.
do not peel
fill cans as full as possible
to each quart add one
teaspoon full of Celery seed
one table spoon each of
Black and white mustard see[d]
than mix ½ cup salt.
1 Pt sugar.
1 Qt Vinegar
1 Pt water
1 cup Olive Oil
this will cover about 5 qts
You can keep them in a
jar if you want to

Wash cucumbers and put in a Jar. mix
2 qts vinegar
1 " Water
1 cup sugar.
1/2 " Mustard
a little Alum.

ICINGS and FILLINGS.

ORANGE FILLING FOR CAKE.

Grated rind and juice of one orange, one-half cup water, one small cup sugar, one teaspoon corn starch, yolks two eggs. Boil, and when cold, put on layers of cake.—Mrs. Frank Payne.

MAPLE FROSTING.

The white of one egg well beaten; boil one cup of maple syrup until it threads; then gradually pour on the egg and beat until it cools.—Mrs. H. Van Allsburg.

CARAMEL FILLING.

One and one-half cups brown sugar, one cup sweet cream; boil slowly until dark and then add the juice of a lemon. Stir until cool, then put in vanilla.—Mrs. O. A. Sears.

FROSTING.

Beat the white of an egg very stiff; place in a bowl in top of the tea kettle and stir in three rounding tablespoonfuls of granulated sugar, stirring until smooth.—Mrs. A. L. Coulter.

CAKE FILLING.

Juice of two lemons and add rind of one, one cup of sugar, three eggs well beaten, one-fourth teaspoonful salt, butter size of egg; boil in double boiler.—Mrs. A. Ross.

CHOCOLATE CREAM ICING FOR LAYER CAKE.

One cup of sugar, one-third cup hot water; put on stove and boil until it spins a thread; then pour it in the beaten white of an egg, and beat until thick enough to spread on the cake. Take half a cup of unsweetened chocolate and melt it in the cup set in boiling water; when melted, spread on top of the icing, and then put the layers together.

CHOCOLATE ICING.

Three-fourths cup of grated chocolate, three-fourths cup of granulated sugar, one tablespoonful cream, one egg. Mix all together; cook in a double boiler until thick, then beat rapidly until cool enough to spread on cake.—Mrs. W. H. Woodley.

NUT FILLING FOR LAYER CAKE.

One cup thick sour cream, one cup sugar, one cup chopped nuts. Stir all together and cook until thick.—Mrs. F. E. Cartier.

MOCHA FILLING.

One cup pulverized sugar, one-half cup butter, soft; one tablespoon cocoa, one teaspoon vanilla, one teaspoon extract coffee. Mix all together until smooth and spread on cake. Make the extract of coffee with one tablespoon of boiling water and two tablespoons of ground coffee.—Mrs. F. H. Hubbard.

COOKIES.

GINGER COOKIES.

Two cups molasses, one cup of sugar, one cup of lard, tablespoonful of soda in a cup of boiling water, salt, tablespoon of ginger, flour enough to roll.—Mrs. Ward.

SOFT GINGER COOKIES.

One cup of molasses, one cup of sugar, one cup of lard, one teaspoonful of salt, one teaspoonful of ginger, two teaspoonfuls of soda dissolved in one cup of hot water. Roll thin; cut in squares and bake quickly.—Mrs. Emma Graves.

HELEN'S MOLASSES COOKIES.

One cup of molasses, one cup of sugar, one egg, one cup of lard, or lard and butter, one tablespoonful of soda, one-half cup of hot water. Flour to mix soft.—Mrs. John Nicholls.

HERMIT COOKIES.

Two cups of brown sugar, one cup molasses, two eggs, one-half cup hot water, salt, one cup lard, one cup raisins, one cup currants, one teaspoonful cinnamon, cloves, nutmeg, one teaspoonful soda. Mix quite hard.—Mrs. F. A. Butler.

MOLASSES COOKIES.

One cup molasses, one cup sugar, one cup lard, one egg, one-half cup of water, one teaspoonful soda, one of ginger, salt. Mix soft.—Mrs. F. A. Butler.

WANDERING JEWS.

One and one-half cups sugar, one cup butter, two cups fruit, one-half teaspoonful soda, one teaspoonful cinnamon and cloves, one-half nutmeg, three eggs.—Mrs. Todd.

HERMITS.

One cup of melted butter (not hot), one and one-half cups light brown sugar, three eggs, one-third teaspoonful of spices, one cup of chopped raisins, one-half cup chopped walnut meats, if desired; one teaspoonful of soda in two tablespoonfuls of cooking molasses, flour sufficient for rolling out desired thickness. Bake in a moderate oven.

MACAROONS.

One pound brown sugar, four eggs, three cups flour, three teaspoonfuls baking powder, one heaping cup cocoanut, one teaspoonful cloves, one teaspoonful cinnamon and a litle salt. Drop on buttered tins and bake in a quick oven.—Mrs. Edyth E. Stacks.

MOLASSES COOKIES.

One cup molasses, one cup sugar, one cup shortening, boil a few minutes. When cool, add one tablespoonful soda, two eggs, salt, ginger, flour to roll thin. Knead thoroughly.—Mrs. Granger.

IDA'S COOKIES.

One and one-half cups sugar, one cup butter, one-half cup sour cream, three eggs beaten one at a time, one teaspoonful of soda in cream, two teaspoonfuls baking powder.—Mrs. O. A. Sears.

WHITE COOKIES.

Two cups sugar, one cup of half butter and half lard, two eggs well beaten, a little nutmeg and salt, one cup sour milk and one teaspoonful soda and one-half teaspoon baking powder in the flour.—Mrs. O. D. Hammond.

SOUR CREAM COOKIES.

Two cups sugar, one cup butter, two eggs, one cup sour cream, one teaspoonful soda dissolved in cream, nutmeg.—Mrs. Will Johnson.

COOKIES.

Two eggs, two cups of sugar, one cup of shortening, one cup of sour milk, one teaspoonful soda, one teaspoonful baking powder, sifted with flour; salt and flavor. Mix soft. —Mrs. Babcock.

CHOCOLATE COOKIES.

Two eggs, two-thirds cup butter, one and one-half cups sugar, one cup grated chocolate, one-half cup sweet milk, two teaspoonfuls baking powder; flour enough to roll out.—Mrs. F. E. Cartier.

WHITE COOKIES.

Two cups sugar, one brown, one white; two eggs, one cup shortening, half lard; one-half cup water, one-half cup sweet milk, two level teaspoons baking powder, one-fourth teaspoon soda. Flavor to taste.—Mrs. Arthur L. Fitch.

SOFT GINGER COOKIES.

One coffee cup shortening, one coffee cup sugar, one coffee cup water, two coffee cups molasses, one tablespoonful soda, one tablespoonful ginger, one teaspoonful salt. Stir stiff with spoon. Roll half-inch thick without moulding, using plenty of flour.—Mrs. Sears.

OATMEAL DROP CAKES.

One cup sugar, one-half cup cream, one-half cup butter, one teaspoonful soda, two eggs, one cup chopped raisins, one teaspoonful cinnamon, one-half teaspoonful salt, two cups flour, two cups rolled oats.—Mrs. A. L. Coulter.

COOKIES.

Two cupfuls brown sugar, three eggs, one cupful shortening, one teaspoonful vanilla, three and one-half tablespoonfuls of sweet milk, one-half teaspoonful soda, a little salt. Mix soft.—Mrs. H. Van Alsburg.

GRAHAM DROP COOKIES.

Two eggs, one cup sugar, one tablespoonful butter, one cup sour milk, one teaspoonful baking powder, one and one-half teaspoonfuls cinnamon, two and one-half cups Graham flour, one cup chopped raisins.—Mrs. M. E. Ackert.

NUT CAKES.

Two eggs beaten light, one cup brown sugar, one scant teacupful of flour, one teaspoonful of baking powder, one-half pound English walnuts. Drop in teaspoonfuls on a greased pan (they spread). Bake in a quick oven.—Edna Sue Green.

MOLASSES COOKIES.

One cup brown sugar, one cup lard, one egg, one cup molasses, one-half cup cold coffee, one heaping teaspoon soda, one teaspoon salt, one-half teaspoon nutmeg, cinnamon and cloves. Mix very soft, roll quite thick; watch closely while baking as they burn easily.—Mary D. Shanahan.

COOKIES.

Sift one quart of flour and one teaspoonful of soda together. Mix thoroughly in this one cup of shortening (one-half butter and one-half lard), then add two cups of sugar. Break two eggs in a cup, beat slightly and fill to the top with sweet milk. When this has been added, mix until of a creamy consistency. Add enough flour to roll out easily.—Olive Hamilton.

HERMITS.

Three eggs beaten, one cup melted butter or other shortening, one and a half cups of brown sugar, one-half cup of molasses, one-half cup of sour milk in which has been stirred a level teaspoon of soda, one cup of cleaned currants, one-half cup of chopped walnut meats, a sifting each of cinnamon, cloves and nutmeg; add three cups of flour. Have a dripping pan well greased, drop a teaspoon of the batter into the pan every two inches apart. The oven should be quite hot when hermits are put in.—Mrs. Harsha.

OATMEAL DROP CAKES.

One cup of sugar, one cup of lard, two eggs, one-half cup of sour milk, one teaspoonful soda, one teaspoonful salt, two and one-half cups of rolled oats, two and one-half cups of flour, three teaspoonfuls cinnamon; fruit if desired. —Mrs. J. Lynn.

ROCKS.

Cream together one cup of butter and one and one-half cups sugar. Add three eggs beaten light, three tablespoonfuls of water, one teaspoonful soda, two and one-half cups flour, measured before sifting, one teaspoonful each of cloves, and cinnamon, one pound of dates, cut fine, and one pound walnuts cut in small pieces. Drop in teaspoonfuls on buttered baking pan and bake in hot oven.

OATMEAL COOKIES.

Two eggs well beaten, one cup melted butter or lard, one and one-half cups of sugar, five tablespoons of sweet milk, three cups of rolled oats, two cups of flour, one cup of raisins, chopped, one teaspoon of cinnamon, one teaspoon of soda.—Mrs. Frank Hull.

WHITE COOKIES.

Two cups of sugar, three-fourths cup of butter, two eggs, one cup of sour cream, one teaspoonful soda level, five cups of sifted flour.—Mrs. Frank Hull.

OAT MEAL CAKES.

One and one-half cups granulated sugar, one-half cup of lard (scant), two eggs, one and one-half cups sour milk, one heaping teaspoonful of soda, one and one-half cups chopped raisins, three large cups of oat meal, salt, flour enough to make a stiff batter, one level teaspoonful of cinnamon.—Mrs. W. H. Woodley.

DROP COOKIES.

One cup sugar, one cup molasses, one cup shortening, two eggs, one teaspoonful ginger, one teaspoon soda dissolved in three tablespoons hot water, two cups flour.—Mrs. John C. Miller.

ORANGE COOKIES.

Two eggs, two cups sugar, one cup butter, six tablespoonfuls sweet milk, three teaspoonfuls baking powder, juice and rind of orange, flour.—Mrs. M. E. Ackert.

GRAHAM DROP CAKES.

One cup sugar, one large tablespoon butter, two eggs well beaten, one and one-half teaspoon cinnamon, one teaspoon soda, two-thirds cup sour milk, one cup chopped raisins, two and one-half cups Graham flour. Dropped on greased tins.—Mrs. H. A. Fowler.

OATMEAL COOKIES.

Two cups brown sugar, three eggs, one cup butter, one cup of lard, ten tablespoonfuls sweet milk, one teaspoonful soda, four cups white flour, four and one-half cups oatmeal, two cups raisins, one teaspoon cinnamon, one teaspoon salt. Mix well together and drop with a spoon.—Mrs. John C. Miller.

GINGER COOKIES

One cup of brown sugar, one cup of molasses, one cup of butter, one-half cup of hot coffee, two eggs, one teaspoonful of ginger, two level teaspoonfuls of soda. Roll soft.—Mrs. W. W. Srigley.

SUGAR COOKIES.

One and one-half cups of sugar, one cup of butter, two eggs, one-half cup of sour cream, one teaspoon of soda. Mix just so you can roll out, then sprinkle with sugar just before putting in oven. Bake quick.—Mrs. F. M. Harris.

OATMEAL COOKIES.

Two cups of flour, two cups of oatmeal, one cup sugar, one cup shortening, one cup sour milk, two teaspoons soda, salt.—Mrs. F. M. Harris.

SOUR CREAM COOKIES.

One cup of butter, one and one-half cups of sugar, three eggs, one cup of sour cream, one teaspoonful soda, two teaspoonfuls baking powder. Flour to make soft dough.—Mrs. Mary Yettaw.

GINGER COOKIES

One cup each of brown sugar, New Orleans cooking molasses and lard. Let come to a good boil, then let partially cool; one teaspoonful each salt and soda, and two teaspoons of ginger, and flour to make very stiff. Keep warm while working.—Mrs. Emily Blodgett.

KILLI-KRANKIES.

Three cups of oatmeal, one teaspoon baking powder, pinch of salt, one cup sugar; mix these together first, then rub in two eggs, one tablespoon melted butter. Mix into little balls size of a walnut, and bake on the bottom of buttered pans.—Mrs. John S. Rood.

CURRANT COOKIES.

Two cups of brown sugar, one cup of shortening, two eggs, one-half cup sour milk, one-half teaspoonful soda, one teaspoonful cinnamon, one teaspoonful allspice, one cup of currants.—Mrs. Mary Yettaw.

MOLASSES COOKIES.

One cup each lard, sugar and New Orleans molasses, two eggs, level teaspoon of cinnamon, heaping teaspoon of soda dissolved in three tablespoons warm water. Work with flour until stiff enough to roll and cut readily; add a little salt. Very nice.—Mrs. Priest.

CHOCOLATE COOKIES.

One cup of sugar, one-half cup of melted butter, one egg, one-half cup of sweet milk, three squares melted chocolate, one and half cups of flour, one-half teaspoonful soda, one and a half cups of nuts and raisins; drop from spoon on buttered tins and bake.—Mrs. J. E. Van Alsburg.

POOR MAN'S COOKIES.

One cup of butter and lard, two cups of sugar, one cup of sour milk, one teaspoonful of soda, two teaspoonfuls baking powder, flour enough to roll quite thin. Any desired flavoring may be added. Very good.—Mrs. E. D. Hines.

MOLASSES COOKIES.

Two cups of molasses, one cup of white sugar, three eggs, one cup of boiling water, two level teaspoonfuls of soda, two teaspoonfuls of baking powder, three eggs, two teaspoonfuls of ginger, salt, one cup of lard and butter. Flour to roll soft.—Mrs. O. A. Sears.

HELEN'S COOKIES.

Two cups of sugar, one cup of butter, one-half teaspoon soda, one cup of sour cream, three eggs beaten separately. Beat cream with yolks. Flour enough to mix soft. Flavor. —Mrs. John Nicholls.

GINGER COOKIES.

One cup of brown sugar, one cup of molasses, one-half cup of sour milk, one-half cup of lard, one teaspoonful of soda, one-half teaspoonful of salt, one dessert spoonful of ginger, cinnamon.—Mrs. W. H. Woodley.

MRS. BARTLETT'S COOKIES.

One-half cup of molasses, one-half cup of brown sugar, one-half cup of shortening, one-half cup of milk, one-half cup Graham flour, one-half cup of white flour, one-half teaspoonful of soda, a little salt. (One-half of the recipe.)

OAT MEAL COOKIES.

Two eggs, one cup of sugar, three-fourths cup of lard and butter mixed, one-half cup of sour milk, two and one-half cups of flour, two and one-half cups of oatmeal, one teaspoonful of soda and a pinch of salt, two level teaspoonfuls of cinnamon.—Mrs. L. E. Benton.

AUNT PHOEBE ANN'S MOLASSES COOKIES.

One cup of molasses, one cup of brown sugar, one cup of shortening, half butter and half dripping, two eggs, two teaspoons of soda, two teaspoons of ginger, pinch of salt. Flour to mix soft. Roll thin.—Mrs. John Nicholls.

WHITE COOKIES.

One cup sugar, two tablespoons butter, two tablespoons lard, two eggs, three tablespoons milk, two teaspoons cream tartar, one teaspoon soda. Enough flour to roll easily. Flavor to taste.—Mrs. Frank Harris.

HERMITS.

One and one-half cups of sugar, one cup of melted butter, three well beaten eggs, one and one-half cups of raisins, one cup of nuts, one-half cup of candied cherries. a little citron, three even cups of flour, two teaspoonfuls of cinnamon, one teaspoonful of cloves, one even teaspoonful of soda dissolved in two tablespoonfuls of water. After all the ingredients have been well beaten, add one teacupful of flour.—Mrs. E. V. Madison.

ANISE COOKIES.

Five eggs, yolks and whites beaten separately; beat yolks with one pound of pulverized sugar; one-half pound of flour with one scant teaspoon of baking powder, two teaspoons of anise seed with whites of eggs beaten in last.—Mrs. Hattie J. Cooper.

MOLASSES COOKIES.

One cup sugar, one cup shortening, two eggs. Cream together. Add one cup cream or sour milk, one-half cup molasses, two teaspoons of soda, one teaspoon ginger, or use any flavoring, salt if needed. Mix soft, and bake in quick oven.—A. Rodger.

HERMITS.

One and one-half cups brown sugar, one cup butter, three eggs, two tablespoonfuls of spices, one teaspoonful of soda dissolved in two tablespoonfuls sour milk, one cup chopped raisins, flour. Chopped nuts may be added, if desired. Cut like cookies and bake in medium oven.—Mrs. A. L. Coulter.

PEPPER NUTS.

One pound sugar, one pound flour, three teaspoons baking powder, four eggs, pinch of salt, one cup chopped nuts, citron and currants to taste. Drop a teaspoonful two inches apart.—Mrs. Marting.

MOLASSES COOKIES.

One cup of molasses, one cup of sugar, one cup of shortening. Boil these together a few minutes, then cool and add one tablespoonful (scant) of soda, two eggs, salt and ginger, two tablespoonfuls vinegar and flour to roll. Mix and knead well. Roll very thin and bake.—Mrs. Granger.

DROP COOKIES.

One-half cup butter, one cup sugar, one egg, one-half cup molasses, one cup sweet milk, one cup raisins, one teaspoon spices, one cup nut meats.—Mrs. Henry B. Wood.

COOKIES.

One and one-half cups of sugar, one cup of butter, one-half cup of sweet milk, two teaspoons of cream tartar sift with the flour, one teaspoonful of soda in the milk, two eggs. Mix soft and bake quickly.—Miss K. L. Meech.

GINGER SNAPS.

Boil one cup of best New Orleans molasses; when cool, add two rounding teaspoons of soda; mix one cup of butter, three-fourths cup of sugar, and two beaten eggs together; then add the molasses and four tablespoons of water, ginger, cinnamon, cloves, allspice. Beat thoroughly and add flour to make a stiff dough; roll thin.—Eva Chamberlain.

COOKIES.

Three cups of flour, one cup of butter, one cup of sugar, one cup of very thick sour cream, one egg, one-half teaspoon of soda. Mix flour, sugar and butter all together. Then make a place in the middle and put cream, soda and egg in; then mix all together. Roll out about one-half inch thick. Flavor with nutmeg and use carraway seed, if desired.—Mrs. F. J. Meech.

RUSSIAN ROCKS.

One and one-half cups of brown sugar, three-fourths cup of butter, three eggs well beaten, one teaspoon of cinnamon, one even teaspoonful of soda in one-half cup of warm water, three cups of flour one cup of raisins, one cup of walnut meats chopped a very little. Drop from a teaspoon.—Mrs. D. F. Meech.

FRIED CAKES.

FRIED CAKES.

One cup sugar, two eggs, five tablespoons melted butter, one cup sour milk, one teaspoon soda, one-half nutmeg. Flour to roll. —Mrs. Mary Yettaw.

FRIED CAKES.

One cup of granulated sugar, one egg, one cup sour milk, one small tablespoon melted lard, small teaspoon soda, one teaspoon baking powder. Add enough flour to roll nicely and fry in hot lard. If you like, add a little grated nutmeg.—Mrs. Wright.

DOUGHNUTS.

One cup of sugar, two eggs, four teaspoonfuls of melted butter; beat together until very light, then add one cup of thick sour milk in which has been dissolved a teaspoonful of soda. Flavor to taste, and add one teaspoonful of baking powder to flour enough to make a soft dough. Fry in the usual way.—Mrs. Rose Taylor.

FRIED CAKES.

One and one-half cups brown sugar, one tablespoonful melted butter, two eggs, one cup buttermilk, one-fourth teaspoonful allspice, three-fourths teaspoonful soda (scant). Just flour enough to roll.—Mrs. Felts.

FRIED CAKES.

One egg, one cup sugar, two tablespoonfuls melted shortening, one cup of sour milk, one teaspoonful soda, nutmeg and little salt.—Mrs. Babcock.

SOUR CREAM FRIED CAKES.

Two eggs, one and one-half cups sugar, one cup sour cream, two-thirds cup sour milk, salt, soda, nutmeg.—Mrs. Will Johnson.

FRIED CAKES.

One heaping cup sugar, two eggs, four tablespoons shortening, one cup sour milk, one heaping spoon soda, salt and any desired flavoring. Roll out quite stiff.—Mrs. L. W. Van Dusen.

DOUGHNUTS.

One cup sugar, two eggs, two tablespoonfuls of melted butter, two-thirds cup of milk, two even teaspoonfuls cream tartar, one even teaspoonful of soda, flour enough to roll, salt and nutmeg. Can use sour milk and soda with as good results.—Mrs. J. H. Reid.

FRIED CAKES.

One cup sugar, two eggs, pinch of salt, one cup sour or buttermilk, a little grated nutmeg, two tablespoonfuls melted butter, one teaspoonful soda sifted in flour. Mix dough as soft as can be handled.—Mrs. Hattie J. Cooper.

FRIED CAKES.

Two eggs, one cup sugar, three tablespoons melted butter, one teaspoon soda dissolved in one cup sour milk, one heaping teaspoon baking powder sifted in enough flour to roll out smoothly. Season with nutmeg. Roll thin and fry in hot lard.—Mrs. Levi Lewis.

FRIED CAKES.

One cupful mashed potatoes, butter size of small walnut; whip to a cream. Beat two eggs lightly. One cup sugar, one-half nutmeg, one-half teaspoonful salt, one-half cup sweet milk, four level teaspoonfuls baking powder.—Mrs. A. D. Cruickshank.

DOUGHNUTS.

Take one cup of sugar and one cup of sweet milk, and mix thoroughly in a bowl and let stand for about fifteen minutes. Then add two well beaten eggs, one teaspoon vanilla, two teaspoons butter, a little nutmeg and two teaspoons baking powder in enough flour to mix and roll out on the board. Fry in lard not too hot, and when done roll in powdered sugar. These are very fine doughnuts.—Mrs. E. King, San Jose, California.

FRUIT FRITTERS.

Make a batter of the yolks of two eggs, one-half cup of water and flour; beat until smooth; add one tablespoonful of melted butter and a little salt; beat again; put in gently the stiffly beaten whites of the two eggs, and set away in the ice box for a couple of hours. Drop into the batter the whole or sliced fruit (you may use almost any kind of fruit), turn each piece until completely covered, and cook in smoking hot fat; drain on rough paper; dust with powdered sugar, and serve hot.—Mrs. J. B. Parsons.

DOUGHNUTS.

One cup sugar and three tablespoonfuls melted lard, well creamed; into this stir well two thoroughly beaten eggs, one cup sour milk, one teaspoonful soda, one teaspoonful baking powder, a pinch of salt, two and one-half cups of flour, or enough to make just stiff enough to handle. Roll out a half inch thick, cut out, and fry in deep fat.—Mrs. W. A. Smith.

DOUGHNUTS.

One cup sugar, two eggs, one cup sour milk, two tablespoonfuls melted lard, one teaspoonful soda, a little nutmeg and vanilla. Mix very soft and fry in hot lard.—Mrs. Le-Fevre.

FRIED CAKES.

One and a half cups of sugar, one cupful of sour milk, two eggs, two scant tablespoonfuls of melted butter, half a nutmeg grated, a large teaspoonful of cinnamon, a teaspoonful of salt, and one of soda. Make a little stiffer than biscuit dough, roll out a quarter of an inch thick and fry in hot lard.—Mrs. Albert Holmes.

FRIED CAKES.

One cup of sugar, four tablespoons of butter, three eggs, one cup of sweet milk, three teaspoons of baking powder, four cups of flour. Roll out one-half inch thick after mixing soft and fry in hot lard.—Mrs. F. J. Meech.

CONSERVES and SAUCES.

Kindly words with fun for spice,
Make a dish that's wondrous nice.

MR JOHN NICHOLLS, adapted tried and guaranteed.

QUINCE HONEY.

One cup grated quince, two and one-half cups sugar, one cup water. Mix well. Cook one-half hour. Bottle and seal. —Mrs. A. T. Burnett.

BECHAMEL SAUCE.

Cook two slices of onion and four of carrot in two tablespoons butter for five minutes, then add one tablespoon flour, one cup water or stock and stir well for two minutes. Add one-half teaspoon salt, one-fourth teaspoon pepper and two unbeaten egg yolks.—Mrs. Marting.

PIE PLANT SAUCE.

Twelve pounds fruit peeled and cut small, twelve pounds sugar, one-fourth pound almond meats, juice of two lemons and peel chopped fine. Let fruit and sugar stand over night. In the morning boil until it thickens, then add the other ingredients, almonds and lemons and two spoonfuls ginger root pounded fine. These last should not be added until ready to take off, then let it stand and heat through and bottle or can.—Mrs. C. L. Judd.

RHUBARB MARMALADE.

Four pounds rhubarb, four oranges, juice of all, peel of two; four pounds sugar, one lemon, two pounds raisins. Cut the rhubarb into half-inch pieces. Prepare the oranges by squeezing out the juice, and cooking the peel of two in water until tender. Drain and scrape out the white part, and chop the yellow peel fine. Extract the juice of the lemon. Put the rhubarb into a preserving kettle. Heat it slowly to boiling, and cook fifteen minutes, then add the sugar, orange juice and peel, lemon juice and raisins, and cook slowly until thick. This is delicious fresh, and a portion may be sealed for future use. One pound of almonds may be blanched and chopped and added the last thing.—Mrs. O. D. Wood.

GRAPE AND APPLE MARMALADE.

To one part apple use two parts of grapes. Cook apples and grapes separately and run through the colander. Add one pint of sugar to one quart of sauce; stir all together, and cook until thick.

QUINCE HONEY.

Three pounds sugar, six large quinces. Place quinces under water when paring. Make the syrup of the sugar. Grate quinces and add every few minutes to boiling syrup. Let boil until thickens. Put in marmalade jars. Delicious. —Mrs. F. M. Sears.

GRAPE CONSERVE.

One pound of raisins, one pound of walnuts, one orange (use both rind and pulp), one basket Concord grapes. Add one cup of sugar to cup and half of fruit. Cook until thick.—Mrs. J. W. Harris.

SPICED CHERRIES.

(A relish with meats.)

Six quarts cherries (pitted), three quarts sugar, one cup vinegar, all kinds of spices. Cook until quite thick. Spiced currants may be prepared in the same manner.—Mrs.Hattie J. Cooper.

ORANGE JELLY.

Three lemons and six oranges. Slice them, but not so fine as for marmalade. Cover with three pints water and let stand twenty-four hours or more, then boil in same water until very tender. Strain through jelly bag. To every cup of juice add one heaping cupful granulated sugar.—Mrs. M. Menzies.

ORANGE MARMALADE.

Take oranges fresh from trees (if you can), cut off each end. Slice very thin with a sharp knife. Cannot be too thin. To each pound of fruit three pints of cold water. Let it stand twenty-four hours. Boil until very soft and set away to stand another twenty-four hours. To every pound of fruit thus prepared, add one and one-fourth pounds of sugar. Boil one hour and forty minutes. Count time from the moment the mixture boils, and make it one hour and forty minutes—no more, no less. Add the juice (not the rind) of one lemon to every three pounds thirty-five minutes before boiling is ended, and when time expires, put into glasses. To hasten jellying, set in the sun.—Mrs. O. D. Wood.

SPICED GOOSEBERRIES.

Three pounds sugar, three pounds fruit, one pint vinegar, one-half ounce cloves, one ounce cinnamon. Boil hard one hour. Bottle and seal.—Miss Emma Bennett.

JIM-JAM JELLY.

One quart of currant juice, one quart of raspberry juice, one pound of seeded raisins, two oranges, five pounds of sugar. It takes about seven pints of raspberries to make a quart of juice. Cook three-fourths of an hour. Chop the rind of the orange very fine; use the whole orange, but be sure no seeds are allowed to remain.—Miss K. L. Meech.

SPICED CURRANTS.

Seven pounds of currants, four pounds of sugar, one-half quart of vinegar, one-half tablespoon of cloves, one heaping tablespoon of cinnamon. Boil one and one-half hours—not longer—as the currants become hard.—Miss K. L. Meech.

PICKLES.

MUSTARD PICKLES.

Mix one-half cup of flour, three tablespoonfuls of mustard, one-half tablespoonful of tumeric, with cold vinegar to smooth the paste. Add three tablespoonfuls of brown sugar and enough vinegar to make a quart in all. Boil until thick and smooth. Have cucumber, onion, cauliflower, green tomatoes and green peppers stand in brine twenty-four hours; scald in brine, then drain thoroughly. Add to mustard and mix thoroughly.—Mrs. H. D. Marshall.

CHOP PICKLES.

One peck green tomatoes, one head cabbage, four large onions, three green peppers, all chopped fine; one cup of salt, one quart of vinegar. Let stand over night and let drain well. Then add three pints of vinegar, four cups brown sugar, one tablespoon each ground mustard, cloves, allspice, cinnamon and ginger, one-half teaspoon each black and red pepper one-half pound of mustard seed. Boil fifteen minutes.—Mrs. Mary Yettaw.

MUSTARD PICKLES.

One green pepper chopped, two quarts little cucumbers, two quarts green tomatoes, two quarts cauliflower, one quart little onions. Soak in salt and water over night. Steam until tender.

Sauce to Pour Over.—One gallon vinegar, one quart brown sugar, two cents worth tumeric powder, two-thirds cup flour wet with vinegar, one-half pound mustard wet with vinegar, salt, one tablespoon ground mixed spices. Cook until it thickens.—Mrs. George Smith.

CHILI SAUCE.

Eighteen large ripe tomatoes, two onions, two red peppers chopped, four cups of vinegar, two tablespoonfuls of salt, four tablespoonfuls of sugar, two tablespoonfuls of cinnamon, two tablespoonfuls of ginger, one tablespoonful of allspice, one-fourth tablespoonful of cloves, one tablespoonful of nutmeg. Boil one hour. Makes three quarts. —Mrs. H. D. Marshall.

GOVERNOR'S SAUCE.

One pound green tomatoes, three green peppers, eight large apples, six onions chopped all together, one and one-half tablespoonfuls of celery seed or one large bunch of celery chopped fine, four cups of vinegar, two or three cups of brown sugar, one or two teaspoonfuls of allspice, cloves, cinnamon, salt to taste.—Mrs. John A. Crawford.

CHILI SAUCE.

Fifty large tomatoes, twelve onions chopped fine, six red peppers, two pounds of brown sugar, eight cups of vinegar, one tablespoon each of ginger, allspice, cloves and cinnamon, six tablespoonfuls of salt. Cook until thick. Scald the vinegar.—Mrs. Jas. Morrison.

CELERY SAUCE.

Fifteen large ripe tomatoes, five large onions, one red pepper, four heads of celery, three and one-half cups vinegar, two tablespoonfuls salt, eight tablespoonfuls sugar. Chop all fine—tomatoes separately. Drain off all the water, then add other ingredients. Cook all together until tender.—Mrs. F. E. Lewis.

SPICED TOMATOES.

Two pounds tomatoes, two pounds sugar, two cups vinegar, one tablespoonful each of cloves, allspice, cinnamon, and one teaspoonful mace. Weigh tomatoes after removing skins. Let tomatoes and sugar simmer for two hours; add rest of the ingredients. Simmer one hour longer, stirring frequently. Seal tightly in cans or bottles.—Mrs. A. L. Coulter.

INDIAN RELISH.

One peck firm, ripe tomatoes skinned, seeded and chopped fine; six onions chopped fine, six green or ripe peppers, chopped; one pint grated horseradish, one quart chopped celery, three tablespoonfuls mustard seed, one-half cupful salt. Dissolve two pounds light brown sugar and two tablespoonfuls of ground cinnamon in two quarts of best cider vinegar; then mix all together cold. Bottle and seal well. Very fine with meats and fish. Will keep for years.—Mrs. G. C. Geiken.

CHILI SAUCE.

Twenty-four tomatoes, six onions, six tablespoonfuls sugar, four tablespoonfuls salt, two tablespoonfuls mustard, two tablespoonfuls all kinds spices, three cups vinegar, two green peppers.—Mrs. M. E. Ackert.

PLUM CATSUP.

Three pounds plums, one and three-fourths pounds sugar, one pint cider vinegar, one tablespoonful cloves, one tablespoonful cinnamon, one tablespoonful pepper and a little salt. Scald plums and put through a colander. Add sugar, spices and vinegar and cook until quite thick.—Mrs. Cartier.

CHOW CHOW.

One peck tomatoes chopped, six large onions chopped, one teacup salt. Stir all together and let it stand over night. Drain well. Take three pints vinegar, three pounds sugar, small tablespoonful each of cloves, cinnamon, ginger, dry mustard, and black pepper. Cook until tender, or about twenty minutes. Stir often, as it burns easily.—Mrs. Will Johnson.

CHILI SAUCE.

Eighteen large tomatoes, six large onions, four chopped red peppers, five teacups of vinegar, six tablespoonfuls of sugar, three tablespoonfuls of salt, one tablespoonful of cinnamon, one tablespoonful of cloves. Boil good one hour.—Mrs. W. W. Srigley.

CUCUMBER PICKLES.

One gallon of vinegar, one cup of salt, one cup of sugar, one cup of mustard, one cup of grated horseradish.—Mrs. W. W. Srigley.

RIPE WATERMELON PICKLE.

Pare the pieces of watermelon and trim, not closely. Boil until tender in salted water. Have ready any sweet pickle syrup boiling and dip from water immediately into syrup and cook until clear. Put away in cans or stone jars. Very nice.—Mrs. J. A. Allen.

BENGAL CHUTNEY.

One pound of brown sugar, one-half pound of salt, one-fourth pound of mustard seed, one-half pound of onions, one ounce of ground ginger, one-half teaspoonful of cayenne pepper, one pound of seeded raisins chopped fine, three pints of vinegar, thirteen large tart apples, nine ripe tomatoes, one-half ounce of tumeric, two teaspoonfuls of ground mustard. Chop all fine, put in a crock and let stand four weeks; stir every day. At the end of four weeks boil five minutes, put back in crock. It will keep all the following summer.—Mrs. John A. Crawford.

MUSTARD PICKLES DRESSING.

Mix one-half cup of flour, three tablespoonfuls of mustard, one-half tablespoonful of tumeric with cold vinegar to a smooth paste. Add three tablespoonfuls of brown sugar and enough vinegar to make a quart in all. Boil until thick and smooth. Make brine and let cucumbers, onion, cauliflower, green tomatoes, green peppers, stand in it twenty-four hours. Scald in the brine and drain thoroughly, then pour the dressing over and let stand.—Mrs. H. D. Marshall.

SPICED GOOSEBERRIES.

Six quarts of gooseberries, green or ripe, nine pounds of sugar, one pint of vinegar, not too strong; one tablespoonful powdered cinnamon, one of cloves, one of allspice. Boil the fruit with one-half the sugar and a little water, one hour and a half. When nearly done, add the rest of the sugar. Set off the stove, and add vinegar and spices.—Mrs. O. D. Wood.

PICKLED PRUNES.

Take four pounds prunes; soak in water two hours, then dry well; lay in stone jar. Now take one quart vinegar, two pounds sugar, two ounces mixed spices; let all this boil one-half hour; then pour over fruit. Repeat this process the following day.—Mrs. H. M. Moos.

COLD MUSTARD PICKLES (Cucumber).

One gallon vinegar, one cup salt, one cup sugar, one cup mustard, one cup horseradish grated or cut in small chunks. Fill jar with cucumbers washed clean, then mix the above, and pour over.—Mrs. D. H. Pierce.

TOMATO CATSUP.

One peck ripe tomatoes cut fine and boil one and one-half hours; add one pound celery, one quart onions, three red peppers, two pounds brown sugar, one-half cup salt, one tablespoon cinnamon, one teaspoon cloves, one teaspoon ground mustard, one quart vinegar. Boil together one-half hour.—Mrs. Chas. Lamoreaux.

PICKLED ONIONS.

Choose small onions. Make brine strong enough to float an egg. When boiling hot, pour over the onions and let them stand for twenty-four hours. Wipe them dry, put into jars; add a small red pepper and a little horseradish. Fill jars with cider vinegar and seal closely.—Mrs. Noble.

CANDY.

WHITE CANDY.

Four cups granulated sugar, two-thirds cup water, and butter the size of a hickory nut, two tablespoonfuls vinegar, one teaspoonful cream of tartar. Boil till crisp, when dropped in water. Do not stir after pouring in the plates to cool, and pour two teaspoonfuls of vanilla over it. Pull as soon as cool enough to handle.—Mrs. O. D. Hammond.

CREAM FUDGE.

Two cups white sugar, three-fourths cup of milk or cream, two squares Baker's chocolate. Cook until it will form soft ball in water. Cook slowly and stir a little. When about done, add butter size of egg. When done, set in pan of cold water until waxy, then stir until thick and turn out. English walnuts improve it.—Caroline Geiken.

COCOANUT SQUARES.

Two cups granulated sugar, one-half cup cream, pinch of salt. Boil, then mix in one-half cup cocoanut. Flavor with teaspoon vanilla.—Caroline Geiken.

FONDANT.

Two cups granulated sugar, one-half or two-thirds cup water, one-eighth teaspoonful cream of tartar. Boil until it hairs or forms a soft ball in water. Pour on greased platter and stir until creamy. Mold with the hands into drops which may be covered with chocolate or flavored with various extracts and nuts pressed on the top.—Mrs. A. L. Coulter.

CREAM MINT.

One pound confectioners' sugar, white of one egg well beaten, two teaspoonfuls ice water, thirty drops oil of peppermint. Mix well, roll on bread board and cut with cutter about size of a quarter.—Mrs. Noble.

FUDGE.

Two cups sugar, one cup milk, one-quarter cake of chocolate, butter one-half size of an egg. Boil until it forms a soft ball in cold water. Let cool; beat thoroughly and pour on greased platter, pressing into shape with the hands.—Mrs. A. L. Coulter.

ORANGE STRAWS.

Cut orange peelings in strips; put them in a granite or porcelain-lined stewpan; cover well with cold water; put on stove and let boil twenty minutes. Drain off the water and repeat twice, making three boilings. Then drain and take as much sugar as peelings, and water enough to make a syrup that will cover. Boil until it hairs, roll in granulated sugar while hot. Place on platter to dry.—Mrs. A. F. Bridge.

BUTTER SCOTCH.

Ingredients.—One cup sugar, one-fourth cup molasses, one tablespoonful vinegar, two tablespoonfuls boiling water, one-half cup butter. Boil all in a granite sauce pan till it will form a ball in cold water, then stir in half a cup of chopped English walnuts and pour into a nice buttered pie plate. When cold, it should be brittle. Crack with quick strokes of a hammer in small pieces.—Alice Anna Bentley.

NUT CREAM FUDGE.

Three cups granulated sugar and one-half cup of rich milk. Boil until a soft ball is formed when tested in cold water. Remove from the fire and add chopped walnuts or finely shredded cocoanut. Stir until creamy. Pour on buttered tins and cut into squares while slightly warm. By adding two teaspoonfuls of cocoa to the sugar and mixing well before adding the milk, the candy is given a chocolate flavor. Cook same as above.

FUDGE.

Two cups sugar, one-half cup milk, one teaspoonful butter, six teaspoonfuls cocoa.—Mrs. Will Johnson.

NUT KISSES.

To the whites of four eggs add one cup granulated sugar, one teaspoonful vanilla and a cup of unbroken nut-meats—hickory nuts, peanuts, almonds or any white-meated nut. Whip the whites until very dry—success depends on this—then add the sugar and vanilla and fold into the eggs lightly; add nuts and put on a paper or inverted pan very quickly, a teaspoonful at a time and into a moderate oven. Bake about one hour, until a golden brown.—Mrs. Robert Davidson.

To keep pancakes from sticking to the griddle without oil on the griddle, put three tablespoonfuls of melted drippings into the batter.

FUDGE.

Three cups of sugar, one cup of milk, two and one-half squares of unsweetened chocolate grated, butter the size of a walnut. Let it boil five minutes after it begins to boil; then beat until it hardens. Spread in square tins; just before it is cold mark off in squares.—Miss K. L. Meech.

PINOCHE.

Four cups of light brown sugar, one cup of rich milk, or if skimmed milk is used, add piece of butter size of walnut. Boil until it will form a firm ball if dropped in cold water. Take off the fire and add one cup of chopped walnut meats and one teaspoon of vanilla. Stir constantly until nearly cold; then spread in buttered tins.—Miss K. L. Meech.

CHAFING DISH RECIPES.

WELSH RAREBIT.

One-half pound fresh cheese, two eggs, one teaspoon melted butter, one-half cup cream, one teaspoon mustard. Pick cheese up with fork, beat the eggs, add the cream, mustard, and cheese, and cook until creamy. Serve on toast.—Mrs. J. L. Crane.

CHEESE OMELET.

Four eggs, four tablespoonfuls milk, walnut of butter, three tablespoonfuls grated cheese. Break the eggs into a bowl with the milk and whip thoroughly. Put the butter in the chafing dish, and when very hot, run the eggs into it; allow it to cook until thick. Use a thin bladed knife to loosen it from the bottom, but do not stir it. When done, carefully roll the edges over until all rolled up. When it begins to thicken, sprinkle the three tablespoonfuls of grated cheese before rolling. Very good..—Pleasant Geiken.

CREAMED CHICKEN.

Two cups cold chicken cut in small pieces, one cup chicken stock, one cup milk or cream, two tablespoonfuls butter, one heaping tablespoonful flour, salt and pepper. Cook the butter and flour together in the chafing dish; add the stock and milk and stir until smooth. Put in the chicken, salt and pepper, and cook three minutes longer.—Caroline Geiken.

FRICASSEE OF DRIED BEEF.

One cup of beef finely chopped, one tablespoonful butter, two eggs, one-half pint of milk. Melt the butter in the milk; add the beef, and cook five minutes, then put in the beaten eggs slowly and stir until the sauce is thick. Serve on toast.—Pleasant Geiken.

DRINKS.

PUNCH.

Four dozen oranges, three dozen lemons, two cans pineapple, one pound candied cherries, sugar to suit the taste. Peel two oranges and cut into dice shape, pineapple the same. Extract the juice from the remaining oranges and lemons; add one tablespoon fruit coloring. Strain before adding diced fruit. Add water to suit the taste. This will serve a large company.—Mrs. A. M. Ross.

RASPBERRY VINEGAR.

One quart berries, in one pint vinegar. Let stand two or three days. Extract juice and to each pint add one pint of sugar. Boil twenty minutes. When cool, bottle.—Miss Emma Bennett.

EGG LEMONADE.

Separate four eggs; beat first the whites, then add the yolks, and beat lightly; dissolve one cup of sugar in a pint of cold water; add to it the juice of four lemons, and then a small quantity of cracked ice. Stir the eggs carefully into this and use at once.—Mrs. A. L. Coulter.

LEMON WHEY.

One cup milk, two tablespoonfuls lemon juice.—Mrs. A. L. Coulter.

HOUSEHOLD HINTS.

To remove iron rust, apply lemon and salt and place in sun. Repeat application until rust disappears.

Flour thrown upon burning oil will immediately extinguish it when water only spreads the flames.

An apple cut and laid in cake box will keep the cake nice and moist and improve rather than injure the flavor.

A little orange peel simmered in fat or butter that is not fresh will remove all unpleasant taste and make it perfectly sweet.

Raw eggs can be made very dainty and delicious by beating separately, adding a little flavoring with sugar to taste to the yolk. Place in a sherbet glass, putting the white with sugar added on the top.—Mrs. F. L. Higbee.

Old potatoes are improved by keeping them in cold water several hours before boiling.

Put salt meat into cold water; fresh meat into boiling water. The more gently meat boils the more tender it is.

Put fish into cold water to boil.

One gallon of ice cream will serve twenty-five persons.

Stale bread or biscuit can be renewed by moistening the top and warming through in the oven.

Fruit stains may be removed from linen by pouring boiling water through the cloth.

Wash ink stains with strong brine and then sponge with lemon juice.

Sponge a grease spot with four tablespoonfuls of alcohol to one of salt.

To dry shoes quickly which have become wet, heat some pebbles in a pan and insert them in the shoes.

Take paint out of clothing by equal parts of ammonia and turpentine.

Rub egg stains on silver with salt on a damp cloth.

To clean mica in stoves, wash in vinegar.

For a burn, apply salt.

For a cut, apply turpentine.

Pour cold water over hard boiled eggs as soon as they are taken from the kettle and they will not be discolored.

Wipe off painted floors and zincs with a cloth wet with kerosene and it will keep them looking bright and fresh.

Hiccough cure: Eat a lump of sugar saturated with vinegar.

Cement for broken china: Take unslacked lime and mix with the white of an egg. This dries quickly.

How to grease a griddle: Use a large piece of beef suet, tied in a cloth.

If the sewing machine runs heavy, cleanse thoroughly with gasoline, then oil.

Use kerosene to clean the sink and bath tub.

When milk boils over, put table salt on immediately to prevent odor.

To easily clean dishes in which food has burned in cooking, soak in warm water to which soda has been added. Cover.

Use a mustard plaster to stop vomiting. Take three teaspoons of mustard with the white of an egg. Place to the throat and stomach.

To renovate silk: Boil kid gloves in water till it becomes a kind of soft glue. Sponge the silk with it, ironing on the wrong side.

Chloroform will take out dried paint stains from cotton or woolen, if butter or olive oil is first applied.

When tired, take a hot salt water bath.

HOW TO COOK A HUSBAND.

Do not go to market for a husband, as the best of them are always brought to your door.

See that the linen in which you wrap him is nicely washed and mended with the required number of buttons well sewed on.

Tie him in the kettle by a strong silk cord called comfort, as the one called duty is apt to be too weak.

Make a clear, steady fire out of love, neatness and cheerfulness, and set him as near this as seems to agree with him. Add a little sugar in the form of what confectioners call kisses, but no vinegar or pepper on any account. A little spice has been known to improve a husband, but must be used sparingly.

Do not stick any sharp instruments into him to see if he is becoming tender. You cannot fail to know when he is done. If cooked in this way, he will keep as long as you want, unless you become careless and set him in too cool a place.

HOW TO PRESERVE A HUSBAND.

Be careful in your selection; do not choose too young and take only such varieties as have been reared in a good moral atmosphere. When once decided upon and selected, let that part remain forever settled, and give your entire thought to preparation for domestic use. Some insist on keeping them in a pickle, while others are constantly getting them into hot water. Even poor varieties may be made sweet, tender and good, by garnishing them with patience, well sweetened smiles, and flavored with kisses to taste; then wrap well in a mantle of charity; keep warm with a steady fire of devotion and serve with peaches and cream. When thus prepared, they will keep for years.—Meconda.

Mary Saunders Rolls

2 tab spoons lard
1/2 cup sugar
1 tab salt
2 cups boiling water
2 well beaten eggs in the soft dough. stir as stiff as possible with flour. let rise. than bake in Muffins tins

CONTENTS.

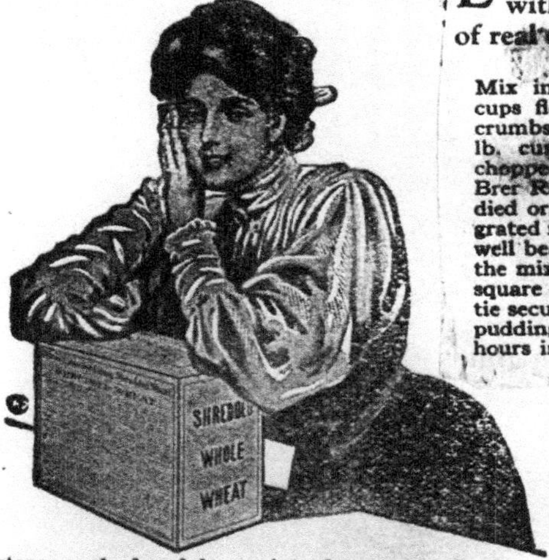

LUSCIOUS made this way—with the longed-for flavor of real old-time molasses:

Mix in the following order 1½ cups flour, 1½ cups stale bread crumbs, ¾ lb. seeded raisins, ¾ lb. currants, ¾ lb. suet finely chopped, 1⅛ cups sugar, 1 cup Brer Rabbit Molasses, 3 ozs. candied orange peel finely cut, 1 tsp. grated nutmeg, 1 tsp. mace, 6 eggs well beaten and 2 tsp. salt. Turn the mixture into a thickly floured square of unbleached cotton cloth, tie securely, allowing room for the pudding to swell, and cook for 5 hours in a kettle of boiling water.

Wheat

for the housekeeper to lean upon in every emergency. Ready-cooked, ready-to-serve, it contains all of the nutritive elements of the whole wheat, steam-cooked and drawn into fine porous shreds so that the stomach may easily take up all its strength-giving properties.

Heated in the oven, Shredded Wheat Biscuit is delicious for breakfast with milk or cream. Recipes for making many wholesome and palatable combinations with fruit or creamed vegetables or meats will be found in this book.

SHREDDED WHEAT BISCUIT and TRISCUIT (the Shredded Wheat Wafer) are made by The Natural Food Company at Niagara Falls in the cleanest and most hygienic food factory in the world. Our new cook book is sent free for the asking.

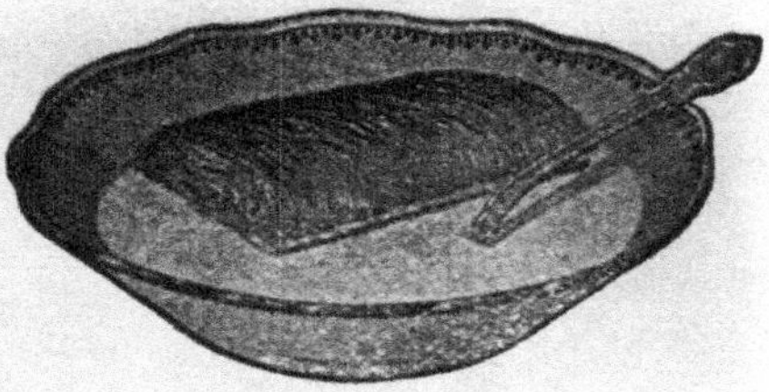

"It's All in the Shreds"

Fire-Life-Accident-Marine-Plate Glass
Steam Boiler-Employers Liability Insurance

MYRTIE YOUNG

Representing
OLD LINE FIRE COMPANIES

Resort property a specialty

Phone 275 *CHARLEVOIX, MICH.*

Made in the USA
Monee, IL
04 November 2026

67378976R00075